I0696876

CARING FOR

DEMENTIA PATIENTS

A step by step guide to making their life safe, happy, and comfortable.

By

Ranulf Hartmann

Copyright © 2023 by Ranulf Hartmann

All rights reserved. No part of this book may be reproduced or transmitted in any form or by any means, electronic or mechanical, including photocopying, recording, or by any information storage and retrieval system, without permission in writing from the publisher.

This book is a work of non-fiction and is intended for informative and educational purposes. Any references to real people, or real places are used in an informative context.

Table of Contents

Introduction

Understanding Dementia

Dementia is a broad term used to describe a group of cognitive disorders characterized by a decline in cognitive function that goes beyond normal aging. It is not a specific disease but a syndrome with a variety of causes, and it primarily affects memory, thinking, behavior, and the ability to perform everyday activities. Dementia is often associated with a progressive and irreversible deterioration in cognitive abilities, and it can significantly impact an individual's quality of life.

Key points to understand about dementia:
¶ Memory Impairment: One of the hallmark symptoms of dementia is memory loss, especially short-term memory. Individuals with dementia may struggle to remember recent events, appointments, or the names of people they know.

¶ Cognitive Decline: Dementia also affects other cognitive functions such as problem-solving, language, attention, and spatial awareness. These deficits can make it challenging for individuals to perform tasks they once managed easily.

¶ Behavioral Changes: Dementia can lead to changes in behavior and personality. Individuals may become more agitated, irritable, or apathetic. Emotional instability and mood swings are common.

¶ Functional Impairment: As dementia progresses, individuals may struggle with activities of daily living, such as dressing, eating, and personal hygiene. They could also have trouble identifying familiar faces or locations.

Types of Dementia

There are various types of dementia, each with its own underlying causes and characteristics. It's important to distinguish between these types because the approach to care and treatment can vary significantly based on the specific form of dementia. A few of the more prevalent kinds are as follows:

1. Alzheimer's Disease: The most common type of dementia is Alzheimer's disease. It is characterized by the accumulation of abnormal protein deposits in the brain, leading to the death of brain cells and cognitive decline. Memory loss and confusion are prominent symptoms in Alzheimer's.

2. Vascular Dementia: This type of dementia is caused by impaired blood flow to the brain, often due to strokes or small vessel disease. It can lead to problems with thinking, reasoning, and memory, and its progression can be stepwise, with distinct episodes of decline.

3. Lewy Body Dementia: This type is characterized by the presence of abnormal protein deposits called Lewy bodies in the brain. It leads to a range of cognitive and motor symptoms, including visual hallucinations, fluctuating alertness, and Parkinson's-like movement issues.

4. Frontotemporal Dementia: This type primarily affects the frontal and temporal lobes of the brain, leading to changes in behavior, personality, and

language abilities. It often occurs at a younger age than Alzheimer's disease.

5. Mixed Dementia: Some individuals may have a combination of different types of dementia, such as Alzheimer's disease and vascular dementia.

6. Other Types: There are rarer forms of dementia, including Creutzfeldt-Jakob disease, Huntington's disease, and more, each with its own unique characteristics and underlying causes.

Understanding the specific type of dementia a person has is crucial for accurate diagnosis, treatment, and planning of care. It also helps caregivers and healthcare professionals tailor their approach to meet the individual's needs and provide the best possible care and support. Additionally, ongoing research is continually expanding our knowledge of the different types of dementia and potential treatments.

Stages of Dementia

Certainly, dementia progresses through several stages, each with its own set of symptoms and challenges. It's important to note that the progression of dementia can vary from person to person, and not everyone will experience all these stages. However, understanding the general stages of dementia can help caregivers and healthcare professionals provide appropriate care and support. The most commonly recognized stages of dementia are as follows:

1. Preclinical Stage:
In the preclinical stage, there are no apparent symptoms of dementia. However, subtle changes in the brain may already be occurring, such as the accumulation of abnormal proteins like amyloid plaques (common in Alzheimer's disease) or vascular changes. These changes may be detected through advanced imaging or biomarker tests, but they do not manifest as noticeable cognitive or functional impairments.

2. Mild Cognitive Impairment (MCI):
MCI is often considered a transitional stage between normal age-related cognitive changes and more severe dementia. People with MCI may experience subtle memory problems or cognitive deficits that

are noticeable to themselves and their loved ones, but these do not yet significantly interfere with daily life or independence. Not everyone with MCI progresses to dementia, and some may remain stable or even improve.

3. Early-Stage Dementia:
At this stage, individuals begin to experience more pronounced cognitive and functional changes, although they can often compensate for these changes with some effort. Common symptoms include:

- Mild memory loss, particularly in regard to recent events.
- Difficulty putting ideas into words or finding the correct words.
- Challenges with organization and planning.
- Mild mood swings or personality changes.

People in the early stage of dementia can often continue to live independently, but they may require more support in certain areas, such as managing finances, transportation, or medication.

4. Middle-Stage Dementia:

The middle stage of dementia is often the longest and can be the most challenging for both individuals with dementia and their caregivers. Symptoms become more pronounced and include:

- Severe memory loss, including difficulty recognizing family and friends.
- Increasing difficulty with communication, leading to frustration and agitation.
- Inability to perform complex tasks, such as cooking or managing finances.
- Wandering and difficulty with spatial orientation.
- Behavioral changes, including mood swings and increased confusion.

Individuals at this stage typically require significant assistance with daily activities and may need to move to a memory care facility or have in-home caregivers to ensure their safety and well-being.

5. Late-Stage Dementia:
In the late stage of dementia, cognitive and physical functions deteriorate significantly. Symptoms include:

- Profound memory loss, including an inability to recognize loved ones or oneself in a mirror.
- Severe communication deficits, often limited to nonverbal expressions.
- Complete dependency on others for all daily needs, including feeding, dressing, and toileting.
- Decline in motor skills and mobility, potentially leading to immobility.
- Vulnerability to infections and other health issues being more prevalent.

Late-stage dementia requires 24/7 care, usually in a specialized care facility or with a team of trained caregivers. Quality of life and comfort become primary concerns, and end-of-life decisions may need to be addressed.

It's important to remember that the progression of dementia is not linear, and individuals may fluctuate between these stages due to various factors. Additionally, the specific symptoms and their severity can vary depending on the type of dementia and the individual's overall health. Caregivers and healthcare professionals play a critical role in providing support and enhancing the quality of life at each stage of dementia.

Chapter 1

The Dementia Care Journey

Caring for a loved one with dementia can be a challenging and emotionally demanding journey. It often begins with the recognition of subtle changes in cognitive function and behavior. Understanding the early signs of dementia is a crucial step in providing appropriate care and support throughout the dementia care journey. This chapter focuses on the initial phase of this journey: recognizing the signs of dementia.

Recognizing the Signs of Dementia

Dementia is a progressive condition, and early detection is key to ensuring individuals receive the best possible care and support. Recognizing the signs of dementia can be challenging, as some of the early symptoms may be subtle and mistaken for normal age-related changes or stress. It's essential to be vigilant and consider the following common symptoms as potential indicators of dementia:

Common Symptoms:

1. Memory Loss: One of the most well-known early signs of dementia is memory impairment. Individuals may have difficulty recalling recent events, names of people they know, or important dates. They may ask the same questions repeatedly or struggle to remember where they placed common items.

2. Difficulty with Planning and Problem-Solving: Dementia can affect an individual's ability to plan and solve problems. They may find it challenging to follow a familiar recipe, manage finances, or complete tasks that involve multiple steps. Frustration and a sense of being lost might result from this.

3. Language and Communication Problems: Individuals with dementia may have trouble finding the right words or expressing their thoughts. They might struggle with understanding conversations or

become repetitive in their speech. This can hinder effective communication and lead to social withdrawal.

4. Disorientation and Confusion: Dementia can cause disorientation, where individuals become confused about time, place, and even their own identity. They may not recognize their surroundings or be unable to differentiate between the past and present.

5. Impaired Judgment: Poor judgment and decision-making can be evident in early dementia. This can manifest in inappropriate social behaviors, financial mistakes, or neglect of personal safety.

6. Mood and Personality Changes: Individuals with dementia may experience mood swings, becoming irritable, anxious, or depressed. Their personality may undergo noticeable shifts, leading to altered behaviors and interests.

7. Difficulty with Familiar Tasks: Dementia can make once-familiar tasks, such as dressing, cooking, or driving, increasingly challenging. Individuals

may struggle with the sequence of steps required for these activities.

8. Social and Occupational Withdrawal: Early-stage dementia can lead to a withdrawal from social activities, hobbies, and work. Individuals may feel overwhelmed by their difficulties and choose to isolate themselves.

9. Loss of Initiative: A lack of initiative or motivation to engage in activities they once enjoyed can be a sign of dementia. Individuals may no longer initiate conversations or participate in their usual hobbies.

Recognizing these common symptoms is the first step in the dementia care journey. If you or someone you know is experiencing these signs, it is crucial to seek a medical evaluation. Early diagnosis allows for effective management, treatment options, and planning for the future. Additionally, it provides an opportunity to access support services and connect with dementia care professionals who can guide you through the complexities of caring for someone with dementia. Remember that a timely and accurate diagnosis can greatly enhance the quality of life for both the individual with dementia and their caregivers.

Early Detection and Diagnosis

Timely detection and diagnosis of dementia are critical for both individuals experiencing cognitive changes and their caregivers. Early intervention can improve the management of the condition, provide access to appropriate resources, and enhance the quality of life for those living with dementia. This section delves into the significance of early detection and diagnosis.

Early Detection and Diagnosis: Why It Matters

¶ Access to Treatment and Support: An early diagnosis allows for the prompt initiation of treatment, which can include medications and interventions that may help slow the progression of certain types of dementia, such as Alzheimer's disease. It also enables individuals and their families to access support services and resources, which can greatly improve the overall care experience.

¶ Improved Quality of Life: With early diagnosis, individuals with dementia and their caregivers can proactively plan for the future. This involves making decisions about healthcare, legal matters, and long-term care options while the individual with dementia can still actively participate in the decision-making process. This can reduce stress and uncertainty for all involved.

¶ Management of Symptoms: Early diagnosis allows for the early management of symptoms. Caregivers and healthcare professionals can implement strategies to address memory loss, communication difficulties, and behavioral changes. This can enhance the individual's ability to function independently for a longer period.

¶ Safety and Well-being: As dementia progresses, individuals may become more susceptible to safety risks, such as wandering, falls, and self-neglect. Early diagnosis enables caregivers to implement safety measures and interventions to minimize these risks, ensuring the well-being of the person with dementia.

¶ Emotional and Psychological Support: An early diagnosis provides an opportunity for individuals with dementia and their caregivers to access emotional and psychological support. This can include counseling, support groups, and education on coping with the emotional impact of dementia.

Chapter 2

Emotional Impact on the Caregiver

Taking care of a loved one who has dementia can be physically and emotionally taxing. The emotional impact on caregivers is profound and often underestimated. Understanding and addressing these emotional challenges is essential for the well-being of caregivers.

Emotional Challenges Faced by Caregivers:

° Grief and Loss: Caregivers often experience a sense of grief and loss as they witness the decline in their loved one's cognitive abilities and personality. It can be emotionally painful to see someone they care for slowly become a different person.

° Stress and Overwhelm: The responsibilities of caregiving can be overwhelming. The demands of providing care, managing household tasks, and balancing one's own life can lead to high levels of stress. Caregivers may feel stretched thin and emotionally drained.

° Feelings of Guilt: Caregivers may experience guilt and self-doubt, questioning whether they are doing enough or making the right decisions for their loved one. This guilt can be especially pronounced when considering decisions about professional care or long-term placement.

° Isolation: Caring for a person with dementia can be isolating. The caregiver's social life and personal pursuits often take a backseat to the demands of caregiving, leading to feelings of loneliness and a lack of support.

° Burnout and Health Issues: Long-term caregiving without adequate self-care can lead to caregiver burnout, which can result in health problems, both physical and emotional.

Addressing the Emotional Impact on Caregivers:

- Consult your friends, family, or support groups for assistance.
- Take breaks to rest and recharge.

- To deal with emotional difficulties, think about counseling or therapy.
- Make self-care a priority by maintaining hobbies and interests.
- Explore respite care options to provide temporary relief for the caregiver.

In conclusion, early detection and diagnosis of dementia are vital for ensuring the best possible care and support for individuals with dementia. Equally important is addressing the emotional impact on caregivers, who play a central role in the dementia care journey. Recognizing and managing the emotional challenges can lead to improved well-being for both individuals with dementia and their dedicated caregivers.

Coping with the Diagnosis

Receiving a dementia diagnosis, whether for yourself or a loved one, can be emotionally overwhelming. It marks the beginning of a challenging journey that affects both the individual with dementia and their caregivers. Coping with the diagnosis is a vital aspect of providing the best possible care and support.

Coping with the Diagnosis

Coping with a dementia diagnosis involves a range of emotional, practical, and psychological adjustments. Here are some strategies and considerations for individuals and caregivers:

* For the Individual with Dementia:

° Understanding and Acceptance: Acknowledging the diagnosis is the first step. Seek information about the specific type of dementia and its progression. Understanding what to expect can help individuals and their families plan for the future.

° Active Engagement: Stay engaged in activities that bring joy and fulfillment. This can include hobbies, creative pursuits, and social interactions. Remaining active and mentally stimulated can slow cognitive decline.

° Building a Support Network: Connect with friends, family, and support groups. Sharing experiences and emotions with others who understand the challenges of dementia can provide a sense of community and comfort.

° Participate in Memory Enhancement Programs: Some individuals find benefit in memory enhancement programs and therapies that help maintain cognitive function and memory skills.

° Legal and Financial Planning: Early planning for legal matters, such as power of attorney and advance directives, can provide individuals with a sense of control over their future.

* For Caregivers:
Coping with the diagnosis is not limited to the individual with dementia; caregivers also face emotional challenges.

Support for Caregivers

Caregivers play a pivotal role in the dementia care journey, and they often need their own support systems to manage the emotional impact of caregiving. Here are ways to find support:

° Support Groups: Joining caregiver support groups can be immensely beneficial. These groups provide a safe space to share experiences, learn from others, and offer emotional support. Many organizations and online platforms offer such groups.

° Professional Guidance: Consider seeking counseling or therapy. A mental health professional can help caregivers process their emotions, manage stress, and develop coping strategies.

° Respite Care: Caregivers need breaks to rest and recharge. Arrange for respite care services, which allow someone else to care for the individual with dementia temporarily, giving caregivers a much-needed break.

° Education: Learn as much as possible about dementia, its stages, and caregiving strategies. Knowledge empowers caregivers and reduces the sense of helplessness.

° Family and Friends: Communicate with your support network. Share your feelings, needs, and challenges with family and friends. They may be willing to provide assistance or simply lend a listening ear.

° Self-Care: Prioritize self-care. It is essential to look after one's physical and mental health. Regular exercise, a balanced diet, and quality sleep are essential for caregivers.

° Set Realistic Expectations: Recognize that you are human and cannot do everything. Setting realistic expectations and boundaries is crucial to prevent burnout.

° Legal and Financial Planning: Plan for the long-term care of the individual with dementia. This includes understanding legal and financial aspects, which can provide caregivers with a sense of security.

° Reach Out to Professional Caregiver Support Services: Many organizations offer caregiver support services that can provide guidance, resources, and respite care.

° Embrace the Moments: While caregiving can be challenging, remember to cherish the moments of connection and love with the person with dementia. Finding joy in small victories and special moments can be emotionally rewarding.

Coping with the diagnosis and providing support for caregivers is an ongoing process. It's critical to keep in mind that asking for assistance and support shows strength rather than weakness. Caregivers and individuals with dementia can navigate this journey with resilience, love, and a strong support network, making the experience as positive as possible given the circumstances.

Chapter 3

Creating a Safe Environment

One of the most critical aspects of caring for individuals with dementia is ensuring their safety and well-being. Creating a safe environment is essential to prevent accidents, injuries, and to promote a sense of security for the person with dementia. In this section, we will focus on home safety for dementia patients.

Home Safety for Dementia Patients

Adapting the home environment to meet the specific needs of individuals with dementia is a crucial part of their care. Dementia can lead to a range of cognitive and physical challenges, making it necessary to make the living space safer. Here are key considerations for home safety:

¶ Reduce Clutter: Clear pathways and living spaces of clutter to minimize tripping hazards. Remove unnecessary furniture, rugs, and objects that can obstruct movement.

¶ Adequate Lighting: Ensure good lighting throughout the home. Poor lighting can lead to confusion and disorientation. Install nightlights in hallways and bathrooms to prevent falls during the night.

¶ Secure Entry and Exit Points: People with dementia may wander. Install locks or alarms on doors and windows to prevent unintended exits. Keyless locks or door alarms can be useful.

¶ Use Childproofing Measures: Childproofing items such as cabinet locks, safety gates, and corner protectors can also be effective in preventing access to potentially harmful objects or areas.

¶ Kitchen Safety: Keep potentially dangerous items out of reach or locked up, such as knives, cleaning products, and stovetop controls. Clearly label cabinets and drawers to help with identification.

¶ Bathroom Safety: Install grab bars in the shower and near the toilet to assist with balance and prevent falls. Non-slip bath mats and shower seats can also enhance safety.

¶ Medication Management: Supervise and manage medications. Use a pill organizer or medication management system to ensure the right doses are taken at the right times. Keep medications locked away to prevent accidental ingestion.

¶ Fire Safety: Check smoke detectors regularly and ensure they are in working order. Create and practice a fire escape plan with the person with dementia and other household members.

¶ Temperature Control: Monitor and regulate room temperatures to prevent overheating or excessive cold. Some individuals with dementia may forget to adjust thermostats or dress appropriately for the weather.

¶ Emergency Contact Information: Place a list of emergency contact numbers, including doctors and family members, in a visible location. Make sure the person with dementia knows where to find it.

¶ Labeling and Signage: Label rooms and key areas of the home with clear, large signage. This can help individuals with dementia recognize different areas and reduce confusion.

¶ Constant Supervision: If necessary, consider 24/7 supervision or in-home care to ensure the individual's safety. Caregivers or professional caregivers can provide the necessary assistance.

¶ Regular Home Safety Checks: Periodically assess the home for safety hazards and make necessary adjustments as the condition of the person with dementia changes.

¶ Wandering Management: Implement strategies to manage wandering behavior, such as providing engaging activities and creating safe wandering spaces within the home or yard.

Creating a safe environment for dementia patients in the home is an ongoing process. As the condition progresses, the safety measures may need to be adapted to meet the changing needs of the individual. Consult with healthcare professionals and organizations specializing in dementia care for guidance on creating the safest possible environment for your loved one. Safety is paramount in providing a comfortable and secure living environment for individuals with dementia.

Preventing Accidents and Falls

Preventing accidents and falls is of paramount importance when caring for individuals with dementia, as they are more prone to injuries due to cognitive and physical impairments. Falls can lead to serious consequences, such as fractures and head injuries. To ensure the safety and well-being of the person with dementia, here are strategies to prevent accidents and falls:

1. Home Modification:

° Remove Tripping Hazards: Clear the home of clutter, including loose rugs, electrical cords, and any objects obstructing pathways.

° Secure Carpets and Rugs: Use non-slip pads or double-sided tape to secure rugs and carpets in place.

° Well-Lit Environment: Ensure proper lighting throughout the house. This includes well-lit hallways, staircases, and bathrooms. Nightlights can be especially helpful in preventing nighttime falls. Install handrails and grab bars in strategic locations, like corridors, bathrooms, and staircases. These aids provide support and stability.

° Secure Furniture: Anchor heavy furniture to the wall to prevent tipping over if the person with dementia attempts to use it for support.

2. Assistive Devices:

° Walking Aids: Consider using walking aids like canes, walkers, or rollators if the person with dementia is prone to balance issues. Ensure these aids are properly fitted and regularly maintained.

° Non-Slip Footwear: Encourage the individual to wear non-slip shoes or slippers with good traction.

Avoid footwear with smooth soles that can increase the risk of slipping.

3. Medication Management:

° Regular Medication Review: Ensure that medications are reviewed by a healthcare professional to identify and mitigate side effects that may increase the risk of falls or dizziness.

° Proper Medication Storage: Keep medications out of reach and locked up to prevent accidental ingestion.

4. Supervision and Monitoring:

° Constant Supervision: If the person with dementia is at high risk for falls, consider 24/7 supervision, especially during nighttime hours.

° Use of Baby Monitors: Baby monitors or motion sensor alarms can be placed in the individual's room to alert caregivers if they get out of bed at night.

5. Exercise and Physical Therapy:

° Strength and Balance Training: Engage the person with dementia in exercises that can improve strength and balance. Physical therapy or occupational therapy may be beneficial in designing appropriate exercises.

6. Cognitive and Sensory Support:

° Cognitive Support: Cognitive training programs can help improve memory and problem-solving skills, reducing the risk of accidents caused by cognitive impairment.

° Sensory Aids: If the person has impaired vision or hearing, provide appropriate aids, such as eyeglasses or hearing aids, to enhance their awareness of their surroundings.

7. Communication and Education:

° Effective Communication: Encourage open communication with the person with dementia about their limitations and the importance of safety. Using clear and simple language can help convey safety instructions.

Educate Caregivers: Ensure that caregivers, both family members and professional caregivers, are well-informed about fall prevention strategies and trained to respond to fall risks.

8. Regular Home Safety Assessments:

Periodically assess the home environment for new fall risks or changes in the person's condition that might necessitate adjustments to the safety measures in place.

Preventing accidents and falls requires a proactive and multifaceted approach. It's important to tailor these strategies to the specific needs and abilities of the person with dementia. Regular communication with healthcare professionals and occupational therapists can provide valuable guidance in implementing effective fall prevention measures and ensuring a safer living environment for individuals with dementia.

Securing Medications and Hazardous Items

Securing medications and hazardous items in the home is an essential aspect of ensuring the safety of individuals with dementia. Cognitive impairment can lead to confusion, forgetfulness, and the risk of accidental ingestion or harm. To prevent such incidents, it is crucial to take specific measures to secure medications and hazardous items:

1. Medication Management:

° Use Medication Organizers: Organize medications using pill dispensers with compartments for different days and times. This helps individuals with dementia and caregivers ensure that the right dose is taken at the right time.

° Store Medications Out of Reach: Keep all medications, including over-the-counter drugs, vitamins, and supplements, in a locked cabinet or box. Make sure it's a location that the person with dementia cannot access independently.

° Medication Monitoring Systems: Consider using electronic medication monitoring systems or automatic pill dispensers with alarms. These devices can provide reminders and help track medication adherence.

◦ Regular Medication Review: Schedule regular medication reviews with healthcare professionals to assess the need for each medication and evaluate potential side effects or interactions.

◦ Proper Disposal: Safely dispose of expired or unused medications, following local guidelines and regulations. This minimizes the risk of accidental ingestion.

2. Securing Hazardous Items:

◦ Lock Cabinets and Drawers: Install childproof locks on cabinets and drawers containing hazardous items. These items can include cleaning supplies, sharp objects, and any potentially harmful substances.

◦ Label Hazardous Items Clearly: Clearly label containers and items with hazardous materials. Use labels with visual cues, as individuals with dementia may struggle to read small print.

° Place Hazardous Items Out of Sight: Store items such as knives, matches, and chemicals in locked or out-of-reach areas. If possible, choose storage areas that are not in the person's line of sight.

° Use Childproof Safety Latches: Install childproof safety latches on toilets, ovens, and other appliances to prevent access to potential dangers.

° Consider Alternative Products: Replace hazardous cleaning products with safer alternatives. For example, use non-toxic, eco-friendly cleaning supplies to reduce the risk of exposure to harmful chemicals.

3. Educate and Supervise:

° Educate the Person with Dementia: Provide education on the dangers of certain items and medications. Use simple language and visual aids to help the individual understand the need for caution.

° Supervise When Necessary: When the person with dementia requires assistance or supervision, make sure that a caregiver or family member is present to monitor their actions and surroundings.

4. Emergency Preparedness:

° Keep Emergency Contact Information Visible: Maintain a list of emergency contacts, including poison control and healthcare providers, in a visible location. Provide clear instructions on what to do in case of accidental ingestion or exposure to hazardous materials.

° Learn Basic First Aid: Caregivers should have basic first aid skills to respond quickly to injuries or accidents. Knowing how to provide immediate care can make a significant difference.

Preventing accidental ingestion or exposure to hazardous items is a critical safety measure when caring for individuals with dementia. Implementing these precautions not only reduces the risk of harm but also provides peace of mind for caregivers and family members. Regular communication with healthcare professionals and occupational therapists can offer further guidance on securing medications and hazardous items in a dementia-friendly environment.

Chapter 4

Wandering and Exit Seeking: Understanding the Behavior

Wandering and exit seeking are common behaviors in individuals with dementia, and they can be distressing for both the person with dementia and their caregivers. Understanding these behaviors is the first step in addressing them effectively.

Wandering:

Wandering involves aimless or repetitive movement within or outside the home. It can be triggered by various factors, including restlessness, anxiety, boredom, a need for exercise, or a response to discomfort or an unmet need. Wandering can become problematic when it poses safety risks, such as wandering outdoors without supervision.

Exit Seeking:

Exit seeking is a subset of wandering where the person with dementia actively seeks to leave a specific area, such as a room or a building. This behavior can be triggered by a desire to return to a familiar place or search for something, often reflecting confusion or a perceived need.

Strategies to Prevent Wandering

Preventing wandering and exit seeking is essential for the safety of individuals with dementia. Consider the following strategies to address and reduce these behaviors:

1. Create a Secure Environment:
* Install locks or alarms on doors and windows: Secure exit points in the home to prevent unsupervised outdoor wandering. Consider devices that provide an alert when a door is opened.

* Implement a secure outdoor area: If available, create a safe outdoor space where the person can wander freely without the risk of leaving the

property. This might include a fenced garden or courtyard.

2. Routine and Engagement:
* Establish a structured daily routine: Consistency in daily activities and schedules can help reduce restlessness and wandering. Meals, exercise, and rest times should be predictable.

* Engage in purposeful activities: Provide the person with dementia with meaningful and engaging activities that reduce boredom and restlessness. These can include hobbies, puzzles, or sensory stimulation.

3. Monitor and Supervise:
* Regular supervision: Ensure that someone is with the person with dementia to monitor their movements and intervene if necessary. This may require assistance from family members, caregivers, or technology (e.g., video monitoring).

* Use motion sensors: Install motion-activated sensors in hallways, doorways, or rooms to alert caregivers when the person starts to move.

4. Communication and Redirection:

* Communication: Engage in clear and empathetic communication. If the person expresses a desire to leave, listen to their concerns and try to address them. Sometimes, explaining that they are safe at home can help.

* Redirection: Offer alternatives or distractions when exit seeking or wandering behavior occurs. Gently guide their attention to a different activity or topic.

5. Identify Triggers:

* Identify potential triggers: Understand what may prompt wandering or exit seeking. It could be hunger, discomfort, the need to use the restroom, or sensory overstimulation. Address these needs promptly.

6. Provide Identification:

* Ensure identification is worn: In case the person does wander away from the home, make sure they have identification with their name and contact information.

7. Medication Management:

* Consult a healthcare professional: If wandering or exit seeking behaviors are extreme or disruptive, discuss the possibility of medication management to address anxiety or restlessness.

8. Wander-Enhancing Environments:
* Create safe wandering spaces: Some individuals benefit from designated wandering areas within the home or an enclosed yard. These spaces should be secure and free from hazards.

9. Professional Support:
* Seek guidance: Consult healthcare professionals or dementia care specialists for personalized strategies and support in managing wandering and exit seeking behaviors.

It's important to approach wandering and exit seeking behaviors with patience and empathy. While preventing these behaviors is crucial for safety, it's equally important to respect the individual's dignity and sense of autonomy. A combination of environmental modifications, engagement, and understanding the person's unique triggers can help manage and reduce these behaviors effectively.

Using Technology for Safety

Technology can play a crucial role in enhancing the safety and well-being of individuals with dementia. It offers various tools and devices that can help caregivers, family members, and the individuals themselves in managing the challenges associated with dementia. Here are some ways technology can be used for safety:

1. GPS Tracking Devices:
*   Wearable GPS Devices: GPS tracking devices, often worn as wristbands or attached to clothing, can help locate the person with dementia if they wander or become lost. These devices provide real-time location information to caregivers or family members.

*   Shoe Insoles: Some GPS tracking insoles fit inside the person's shoes and provide discreet tracking capabilities. They can be especially useful for individuals who remove wristbands or other devices.

2. Home Monitoring and Security Systems:
* Video Cameras: Video monitoring systems can be installed to keep an eye on the individual's movements within the home. This can provide peace of mind to caregivers and help ensure safety.

* Motion Sensors: Motion-activated sensors placed in doorways and hallways can alert caregivers when the person is on the move. These sensors can trigger alarms or notifications.

* Door and Window Alarms: Install alarms on doors and windows to notify caregivers or family members if they are opened. These systems can prevent exit-seeking behavior.

3. Medication Management Systems:
* Automatic Pill Dispensers: These devices can be programmed to dispense medications at specific times, reducing the risk of missed doses. Some models can even send notifications to caregivers if a dose is missed.

4. Medical Alert Systems:

* Personal Emergency Response Systems (PERS): These wearable devices allow individuals to call for help in case of an emergency by pressing a button. Caregivers or emergency services are alerted when assistance is needed.

5. Smartphone Apps:
* Dementia Care Apps: There are numerous smartphone apps designed to assist caregivers and individuals with dementia. These apps can help manage schedules, provide medication reminders, and offer safety tips.

* Locating Apps: Smartphone apps that utilize GPS technology can help locate a missing person quickly. Such apps can be invaluable in the event the individual becomes lost.

6. Medication Reminder Apps:
* Medication Reminder Apps: Various apps are available for smartphones and tablets that provide medication reminders and help track medication schedules. They can be particularly helpful for both individuals with dementia and caregivers.

7. Home Automation and Smart Devices:

* Smart Thermostats and Lighting: Smart home devices can be programmed to maintain a comfortable environment within the home. For example, smart thermostats can regulate temperature, and smart lighting can provide adequate lighting during nighttime hours.

8. Communication and Entertainment:
* Tablets and Communication Apps: Tablets can be loaded with communication apps to help individuals with dementia express their needs and communicate with caregivers or family members.

* Entertainment Apps: Tablets and devices can also offer entertainment options, including games, music, and video content, which can help reduce boredom and restlessness.

9. Remote Caregiver Monitoring:
* Telehealth and Remote Monitoring: Telehealth services and remote monitoring technologies allow healthcare professionals to assess the person's well-being from a distance. These tools can provide valuable insights into the individual's health and safety.

Using technology for safety in dementia care is a valuable tool, but it's essential to select and implement the appropriate solutions based on the individual's specific needs and abilities. Consultation with healthcare professionals and experts in dementia care can provide guidance on the most suitable technology solutions to enhance safety and quality of life for individuals with dementia.

Chapter 5

Providing Daily Care

Caring for individuals with dementia requires a well-structured daily routine that provides stability, promotes a sense of security, and minimizes anxiety and confusion. Establishing a daily routine is essential for the well-being of the person with dementia and can make the caregiving process more manageable. Here are some key considerations when developing a daily routine for dementia care:

1. Consistency:
* Maintain Regular Times: Establish set times for daily activities such as waking up, meals, bathing, and bedtime. Consistency helps individuals with dementia know what to expect and reduces stress.

* Consistent Caregivers: Whenever possible, aim for consistent caregiving personnel. Familiar faces can provide comfort and reduce agitation.

2. Simplicity:

* Simplify Tasks: Break down daily tasks into simple, manageable steps. When giving directions, use terms that are straightforward and simple.

* Reduce Choices: Offer limited choices to avoid overwhelming the person with dementia. Instead of asking, "What would you like for breakfast?" for instance. you can say, "It's time for breakfast. Would you like cereal or toast today?"

3. Promote Independence:
* Encourage Self-Care: Encourage the individual to perform tasks they can manage independently. This enhances one's feeling of self-worth and accomplishment.

* Provide Assistance as Needed: Be prepared to assist when necessary. Offer guidance and support with patience, allowing them to do as much as they can by themselves.

4. Structured Activities:
* Engage in Purposeful Activities: Plan activities that are enjoyable and stimulate the person's mind. These can include hobbies, simple games, art, or

listening to music. Engaging in activities can reduce boredom and restlessness.

* Physical Exercise: Include daily physical activity appropriate to the individual's abilities. Even a short walk or gentle stretching exercises can be beneficial for maintaining mobility and well-being.

5. Mealtime Management:
* Balanced Diet: Ensure that meals are well-balanced and that dietary restrictions or preferences are respected. Maintain regular mealtimes to prevent confusion about when to eat.

* Assist with Eating: Be prepared to assist with eating if necessary. Ensure a comfortable and supportive eating environment.

6. Communication and Interaction:
* Maintain Conversation: Engage in regular conversation to maintain social connections. Even if the person has difficulty with verbal communication, active listening and non-verbal communication can foster a sense of connection.

* Cue Card or Visual Schedule: Use visual cues or cue cards to help the individual understand the daily routine. These cues can include pictures or simple text that illustrate each activity.

7. Manage Sleep Patterns:
* Establish a Bedtime Routine: Create a bedtime routine that promotes relaxation and signals the end of the day. This can include activities like reading a book, gentle stretching, or listening to calming music.

* Minimize Daytime Naps: Encourage daytime activity to reduce excessive napping, which can disrupt nighttime sleep.

8. Flexibility:
* Be Adaptable: While routines are crucial, it's also important to be flexible. Dementia care involves being responsive to changing needs and emotions.

* Monitor and Adjust: Regularly assess the effectiveness of the routine and make adjustments as necessary. Over time, a person suffering from dementia may have different demands and capacities.

Developing a daily routine for dementia care is a dynamic process that requires patience and adaptability. It should be tailored to the individual's specific needs, abilities, and preferences. Regular communication with healthcare professionals, occupational therapists, and other experts in dementia care can provide valuable insights and guidance in creating a routine that best suits the person's well-being and quality of life.

Structured Activities for Dementia Care

Structured activities are an essential component of dementia care, providing individuals with cognitive stimulation, social engagement, and a sense of purpose. These activities can enhance the quality of life for individuals with dementia and offer numerous benefits for their well-being. Here are some key considerations when planning and implementing structured activities:

1. Benefits of Structured Activities:

* Cognitive Stimulation: Structured activities engage the mind, which can help maintain cognitive abilities and slow cognitive decline in some cases.

* Emotional Well-Being: Meaningful activities can evoke positive emotions, reduce anxiety, and combat feelings of boredom or restlessness.

* Social Interaction: Activities that involve interaction with others foster social engagement and reduce feelings of isolation.

* Routine and Predictability: Structured activities contribute to a sense of routine and predictability, which can reduce confusion and anxiety.

* Sense of Achievement: Completing tasks and activities can provide individuals with a sense of accomplishment and boost self-esteem.

2. Planning Structured Activities:
* Tailor Activities to the Individual: Consider the person's interests, hobbies, and past experiences. Activities that align with their previous preferences are often most engaging.

* Vary Activities: Include a variety of activities to keep the person engaged and prevent boredom. This might involve a mix of cognitive, physical, and creative activities.

* Adapt as Needed: Be flexible and adjust activities based on the individual's current abilities. Modify activities to ensure they are achievable and enjoyable.

* Schedule Activities: Integrate structured activities into the daily routine. Consistent scheduling helps individuals know what to expect.

3. Types of Structured Activities:
* Cognitive Activities: These can include puzzles, memory games, word games, and reading. Cognitive activities stimulate the mind and can be adapted to various levels of cognitive function.

* Physical Activities: Gentle exercises, yoga, or even taking short walks can promote physical well-being. Modify these activities to the individual's physical capabilities.

* Arts and Crafts: Creative activities like drawing, painting, or crafting can provide a creative outlet and a sense of achievement.

* Music and Singing: Listening to music, playing musical instruments, or participating in group sing-alongs can be emotionally enriching.

* Cooking and Baking: Simple cooking or baking activities can be both enjoyable and practical. They can engage the senses and stimulate memories.

* Gardening: Gardening activities, whether indoors or outdoors, allow for a connection with nature and a sense of accomplishment.

* Reminiscence Activities: Looking at old photos, sharing stories, or using memory books can help individuals reconnect with their past and share meaningful experiences.

4. Communication and Interaction:
* Engage in Conversation: Communicate with the individual during activities. Encourage conversation and active listening.

* Use Visual Aids: Visual cues or props can make activities more accessible and help individuals understand instructions.

* Group Activities: Group activities, if possible, encourage social interaction. These can be especially meaningful in a care facility or when multiple family members are involved in caregiving.

5. Safety and Supervision:
* Ensure the environment is safe and free from hazards during activities. Consider the individual's physical limitations and adapt the space accordingly.

* Provide supervision and assistance as needed to ensure safety and support participation.

6. Monitor and Adjust:
* Regularly assess the effectiveness of structured activities and make adjustments based on the individual's changing needs and abilities.

Structured activities are a valuable tool in dementia care, and they can be an enriching and fulfilling part of an individual's daily life. By incorporating a variety of activities that align with the person's interests and abilities, caregivers can enhance the well-being and quality of life for individuals living with dementia.

Meal Planning and Nutrition in Dementia Care

Proper meal planning and nutrition are essential aspects of caring for individuals with dementia. As cognitive and physical changes progress, maintaining a well-balanced diet becomes increasingly important for their overall health and well-being. Here are key considerations when it comes to meal planning and nutrition in dementia care:

1. The Importance of Nutrition:
* Nutrient-Rich Diet: Individuals with dementia should have access to a balanced diet that provides essential nutrients. Adequate nutrition is crucial for maintaining physical health and cognitive function.
* Hydration: Ensure that the person stays well-hydrated, as dehydration can exacerbate confusion and other dementia symptoms. Encourage regular fluid intake.

2. Meal Planning:
* Regular Meal Schedule: Establish a routine for meal times. Consistent meal schedules can help reduce confusion and anxiety.

* Balanced Meals: Plan meals that include a variety of foods from all food groups, including fruits, vegetables, whole grains, lean proteins, and dairy products or alternatives.

* Portion Control: Monitor portion sizes to prevent overeating or undereating. Individuals with dementia may not recognize when they are full or may forget to eat.

3. Addressing Dietary Preferences:
* Respect Food Preferences: Consider the person's food preferences and dietary restrictions. Respect their choices while ensuring they receive adequate nutrition.

* Familiar Foods: Sometimes individuals with dementia may prefer familiar foods. Include comfort foods that they enjoy to encourage eating.

4. Texture-Modified Diets:
* Soft and Pureed Diets: For individuals with swallowing difficulties, consult a healthcare professional for guidance on texture-modified diets. These diets can help reduce the risk of choking.

5. Supervision and Assistance:
* Provide Assistance: Depending on the individual's abilities, they may require assistance with meal preparation, setting the table, and eating. Be patient and supportive.

* Cue Cards: Use visual cues or cue cards with images or simple text to help the person understand mealtime steps. This can be particularly helpful for individuals with communication difficulties.

6. Reduce Distractions:
* Minimize Distractions: Create a calm and quiet eating environment. Reduce distractions, such as excessive noise or television, which can disrupt mealtime focus.

7. Special Considerations:
* Chewing and Swallowing Issues: Pay attention to any difficulties with chewing or swallowing.

Consult a speech therapist or healthcare professional for guidance on managing these issues.

* Dental Health: Ensure that the person's oral health is maintained. Regular dental check-ups are essential, as dental problems can affect eating and nutrition.

8. Supervise and Monitor Dietary Changes:
* Weight and Nutritional Monitoring: Keep track of the individual's weight and nutritional intake. If there are significant changes, consult a healthcare professional for guidance.

* Monitor for Food Allergies: Be aware of any food allergies or sensitivities, and make necessary adjustments to the diet.

9. Familiarity and Comfort:
* Structured Mealtime Routine: Establish a structured mealtime routine to promote familiarity and comfort. The routine can include setting the table, washing hands, and saying grace if that's part of the person's tradition.

* Maintain Family Traditions: Continue to celebrate family traditions and special occasions involving food to create a sense of continuity and connection.

10. Emotional Aspects:
* Emotional Well-Being: Mealtime should be a positive and enjoyable experience. Engage in pleasant conversation and maintain a relaxed atmosphere.

* Encourage Independence: Whenever possible, allow the individual to eat independently. Encourage them to use utensils and drink from a cup if they can.

11. Consult a Dietitian or Nutritionist:
A registered dietitian or nutritionist can provide personalized recommendations for meal planning based on the individual's specific dietary needs and preferences.

Proper meal planning and nutrition in dementia care help ensure that individuals receive the nourishment they need to maintain their health and well-being. It's essential to approach mealtime with patience, respect, and sensitivity to the individual's preferences and abilities. Regular communication with healthcare professionals and dietary experts can provide valuable guidance in addressing the unique nutritional needs of individuals with dementia.

Chapter 6

Personal Care and Hygiene

Maintaining good personal care and hygiene is essential for the well-being and dignity of individuals with dementia. As the condition progresses, they may require increasing assistance with activities of daily living. This section focuses on bathing and dressing, two fundamental aspects of personal care for individuals with dementia.

Bathing and Dressing

Bathing and dressing can be challenging for individuals with dementia due to cognitive and physical changes. Caregivers need to approach these tasks with sensitivity and patience to ensure the person's comfort and dignity.

Bathing:
* Establish a Routine: Creating a consistent bathing schedule can help the person with dementia become

more comfortable with the process. Choose a time when they are most alert and relaxed.

* Maintain a Calm Environment: Ensure the bathroom is well-lit and at a comfortable temperature. Remove clutter and any potential hazards.

* Use Visual Cues: Visual cues, such as a picture of a bathtub or shower, can help the person understand the upcoming activity and reduce anxiety.

* Provide Choices: Offer choices when appropriate. For example, ask if they prefer a bath or a shower, or if they would like a specific soap or shampoo.

* Use Gentle and Clear Communication: Speak in a calm and reassuring manner. Explain each step of the process before and as you go along. Use simple and concise instructions.

* Ensure Privacy: Respect the person's privacy and dignity during the bathing process. Use towels or bathrobes strategically to cover areas that may make them uncomfortable.

* Safety Precautions: Use non-slip bath mats in the tub or shower to prevent falls. Handrails and grab bars can provide support when getting in and out.

Dressing:

* Simplify Clothing Choices: Lay out a limited number of clothing options to avoid overwhelming choices. Choose clothing that is easy to put on and take off, with large buttons or zippers.

* Break Down the Process: Instead of handing the person a complete outfit, break down dressing into steps. For example, hand them one item at a time (e.g., socks, pants, shirt) and provide assistance as needed.

* Use Adaptive Clothing: Adaptive clothing, such as garments with Velcro closures or elastic waistbands, can make dressing more manageable for individuals with limited dexterity.

* Respect Independence: Encourage the person to do as much as they can independently. Even if they can only manage one small step, it can provide a sense of accomplishment.

* Assist with Patience: Offer gentle assistance, and maintain a calm and unhurried pace. Give the individual time to cooperate and participate in the dressing process.

* Check for Comfort: Ensure that clothing is comfortable and suitable for the weather. Pay attention to details like socks and shoes, which can impact comfort and balance.

* Use Visual Prompts: If necessary, provide visual prompts to help the person understand the dressing sequence. Visual cues, such as a picture of socks being put on, can be helpful.

* Respect Personal Preferences: If the person insists on wearing a specific item of clothing, prioritize their comfort and choices when possible.

Bathing and dressing can be sensitive areas for individuals with dementia, and maintaining their dignity and comfort is essential. Caregivers should adapt their approach based on the individual's specific needs and abilities. Patience, clear communication, and a focus on maintaining independence can significantly improve the experience for both the person with dementia and their caregiver.

Dental and Skin Care in Dementia Care

Dental and skin care are important components of overall well-being for individuals with dementia. As cognitive and physical changes progress, maintaining good oral hygiene and skin health becomes increasingly important. Here are key considerations when it comes to dental and skin care in dementia care:

Dental Care:

1. Oral Hygiene:
* Regular Brushing: Encourage regular brushing of teeth. Use a soft-bristle toothbrush and fluoride toothpaste. Be gentle and patient during the process.

* Assistance with Brushing: In cases where the person with dementia cannot brush their teeth independently, provide assistance. Ensure that toothbrushes and toothpaste are readily available.

* Flossing: Depending on the individual's abilities, flossing can help prevent gum disease and cavities. Consult a dentist or dental hygienist for guidance on proper technique.

2. Dental Check-Ups:
* Regular Dental Visits: Schedule regular dental check-ups and cleanings to maintain oral health. Inform the dentist about the individual's dementia so that they can provide appropriate care.

* Specialized Dentists: In some cases, a dentist with experience in geriatric or special care dentistry may be best equipped to address the unique needs of individuals with dementia.

3. Denture Care:
* Clean Dentures: If the person with dementia wears dentures, ensure they are cleaned daily to prevent infections and discomfort.

* Proper Fit: Regularly check the fit of dentures, as changes in jaw alignment can occur. Ill-fitting dentures can lead to sore spots and difficulty eating.

4. Address Dental Pain and Discomfort:
* Monitor for Pain: Individuals with dementia may not always express when they are in pain. Watch for signs of oral discomfort or difficulty eating.

* Use Pain Relief as Needed: If dental issues or pain are identified, consult a dentist for appropriate pain management and treatment.

Skin Care:

1. Skin Hygiene:
* Regular Bathing: Ensure that the person with dementia bathes regularly to maintain skin hygiene. Use gentle, moisturizing soaps and lukewarm water.

* Moisturize: Apply a gentle, hypoallergenic moisturizer to prevent dry skin. Give particular care to dry spots like the elbows and knees.

* Skin Inspection: Regularly inspect the skin for signs of irritation, pressure sores, or skin conditions. Promptly address any issues that arise.

2. Pressure Sore Prevention:

* Repositioning: If the person is bedridden or spends extended periods in a chair, reposition them regularly to prevent pressure sores. Use pressure-relieving cushions or mattresses when needed.

* Nutrition: Adequate nutrition plays a role in skin health. Ensure that the individual receives a well-balanced diet to support skin maintenance.

3. Sun Protection:
* Sunscreen: Apply sunscreen when the person is exposed to direct sunlight. Protecting the skin from the sun is essential to prevent sunburn and skin damage.

4. Wound Care:
* Prompt Attention: If wounds, cuts, or bruises occur, provide prompt and appropriate care. Keep wounds clean and apply bandages as needed.

5. Consult a Dermatologist:
If the person with dementia develops skin conditions, consult a dermatologist for specialized guidance and treatment.

Proper dental and skin care in dementia care contribute to overall health and well-being. It's important to approach these aspects of care with sensitivity and patience. Regular communication with healthcare professionals, including dentists and dermatologists, can provide valuable guidance in addressing the unique dental and skin care needs of individuals with dementia.

Chapter 7

Enhancing Communication in Dementia Care

Communication is a fundamental aspect of providing quality care for individuals with dementia. As the condition progresses, it can lead to significant challenges in understanding and expressing thoughts and emotions. However, there are strategies and techniques that can enhance communication and improve the quality of life for both the person with dementia and their caregivers.

Communication Challenges in Dementia:

Understanding the communication challenges in dementia is essential for implementing effective strategies. Here are some of the common issues that individuals with dementia may face:

* Difficulty Finding Words: Many individuals with dementia struggle to find the right words to express

themselves. This can lead to frustration and communication breakdowns.

* Memory Impairment: Short-term memory loss is common in dementia, making it challenging to remember recent conversations or events.

* Repetitive Communication: Individuals with dementia may repeat questions or statements due to forgetfulness or an inability to recall previous conversations.

* Difficulty Understanding: Processing and comprehending spoken language can become increasingly challenging, leading to misunderstandings.

* Emotional Changes: Dementia can lead to emotional fluctuations, making it difficult to convey emotions effectively.

* Non-Verbal Communication: Dementia can impact non-verbal communication, including facial expressions and body language, making it harder to interpret emotions and intentions.

Non-Verbal Communication in Dementia Care

Non-verbal communication plays a critical role in dementia care, especially as the ability to express thoughts and emotions through verbal language declines. Understanding and effectively using non-verbal cues are essential for caregivers and family members to connect with and provide care for individuals with dementia. Here are key aspects of non-verbal communication in dementia care:

1. Importance of Non-Verbal Communication:

* Alternative Means of Expression: As verbal communication abilities deteriorate in dementia, non-verbal communication becomes a primary means of conveying emotions, needs, and intentions.

* Building Connections: Non-verbal cues allow individuals with dementia to connect with caregivers, family members, and peers, even when spoken language is limited.

2. Types of Non-Verbal Communication:

* Facial Expressions: The face is an excellent tool for communicating emotions. Pay attention to smiles, frowns, raised eyebrows, and other facial expressions to understand the person's feelings.

* Gestures: Hand movements, pointing, and other gestures can communicate needs, preferences, and reactions.

* Eye Contact: Maintain eye contact to convey interest and establish a connection during conversations.

* Body Language: Body posture, stance, and movements provide valuable insights into the person's comfort, discomfort, or emotional state.

* Tone of Voice: Although not strictly non-verbal, the tone and pitch of the voice can convey emotions and intentions.

* Touch: Physical touch, such as holding hands or a comforting pat on the shoulder, can convey care, support, and affection.

3. Interpreting Non-Verbal Cues:

* Observation: To understand non-verbal cues, keen observation is essential. Pay attention to changes in facial expressions, gestures, and body language.

* Context: Non-verbal cues are often context-dependent. Consider the situation, environment, and recent events to interpret non-verbal communication accurately.

* Validation: When you interpret a non-verbal cue, validate the person's feelings by acknowledging their emotions or needs. This includes phrases such, "I see you're upset," or "You seem happy today."

4. Effective Use of Non-Verbal Communication:

* Be Present: Give the person your full attention when they communicate non-verbally. This shows that you respect and care for their feelings.

* Respond Appropriately: Respond to non-verbal cues with empathy and care. Offer support or assistance when needed, and adjust your actions based on the cues you perceive.

* Use Non-Verbal Cues Yourself: Non-verbal communication goes both ways. Use gestures, facial expressions, and body language to convey warmth, understanding, and support.

5. Non-Verbal Communication for Comfort:

* Provide Reassurance: Use non-verbal cues to reassure and comfort the person when they are upset or anxious. A gentle touch or a comforting expression can go a long way.

* Non-Verbal Validation: Sometimes, individuals with dementia may struggle to express themselves verbally. You can use non-verbal cues to validate their emotions by mirroring their expressions or using gestures.

6. Tailoring Non-Verbal Communication:

* Adapt to Individual Needs: Different individuals may respond differently to non-verbal cues. It's essential to adapt your communication style to the specific preferences and comfort level of the person with dementia.

* Respect Personal Space: Be mindful of personal space and physical boundaries, as individuals with dementia may have varying comfort levels with touch and physical proximity.

Non-verbal communication is a powerful tool in dementia care, enabling individuals with limited verbal abilities to express themselves and connect with their caregivers. By being attentive, empathetic, and responsive to non-verbal cues, caregivers and family members can create a supportive and comforting environment that enhances the well-being of individuals with dementia.

Strategies for Effective Communication in Dementia Care

Effective communication is at the heart of providing quality care for individuals with dementia. As the condition progresses, the ability to express thoughts and emotions through verbal language may diminish. To maintain meaningful connections and ensure the well-being of individuals with dementia, caregivers and family members must employ a range of strategies for effective communication. Here are comprehensive strategies for effective communication in dementia care:

1. Use Clear and Simple Language:
* Speak Slowly and Clearly: Enunciate words clearly and maintain a moderate pace when speaking. Refrain from using complicated jargon or speaking too hastily.

* Short Sentences: Use short, straightforward sentences to convey information and instructions. Avoid long, convoluted explanations.

2. Maintain Eye Contact:
* Establish Connection: Maintain eye contact to establish a connection and convey interest. Eye contact can help individuals feel acknowledged and respected.

3. Active Listening:

* Pay Attention: Listen actively and attentively to the person with dementia. Demonstrate your sincere interest in what they have to say.

* Avoid Interrupting: Give the person time to express themselves without interruption. Avoid the urge to finish their sentences.

4. Use Visual Aids:
* Visual Cues: Utilize visual aids, such as pictures, diagrams, or written notes, to support verbal communication. Visual cues can clarify information and facilitate understanding.

5. Encourage Non-Verbal Communication:
* Gestures: Be attentive to gestures and non-verbal cues used by the person with dementia. Respond to these cues as they can provide valuable insights into their needs and emotions.

* Facial Expressions: Observe and interpret facial expressions, as they often convey emotions or reactions when verbal language is limited.

6. Be Patient and Empathetic:
* Maintain Patience: Recognize that individuals with dementia may require extra time to process information and respond. Avoid showing frustration or impatience.

*   Empathize: Put yourself in the person's shoes to understand their emotions and perspective. Respond with compassion and understanding.

7. Encourage Communication:
* Open-Ended Questions: Ask open-ended questions that encourage conversation and allow the person to express themselves. Open-ended questions typically begin with phrases like "What," "How," or "Tell me about."

*   Prompt Memories: Use prompts related to the person's past or interests to initiate conversations. Memory cues can stimulate reminiscence and communication.

8. Minimize Distractions:
*   Quiet Environment: Create a quiet and distraction-free environment for conversations. Reduce background noise and visual stimuli that may disrupt communication.

9. Provide Choices:
* Empower with Choices: Whenever possible, offer choices to the person to provide a sense of control.

Ask them, "Would you like tea or coffee?" for instance. instead of making unilateral decisions.

10. Redirect and Reframe:
* Avoid Correcting: If the person says something that is factually incorrect or nonsensical, avoid correcting them. Instead, focus on understanding their intention and feelings.

* Rephrase and Redirect: If the person becomes agitated or confused, rephrase questions or statements to simplify the conversation. Redirect the discussion to a more positive or calming topic.

11. Reinforce Positive Behavior:
* Positive Feedback: Provide positive reinforcement for effective communication. Praise the person for their efforts to engage in conversation.

12. Maintain Routine:
* Consistent Schedule: Maintain a consistent routine for daily activities and conversations. Predictability can reduce anxiety and improve communication.

13. Seek Professional Support:

* Speech Therapy: Consult a speech therapist who specializes in dementia care for personalized guidance on communication strategies.

14. Family and Caregiver Communication:
* Consistency: Ensure that all family members and caregivers use consistent communication strategies to avoid confusion and frustration for the individual with dementia.

15. Be Flexible:
* Adapt Communication: Be adaptable and open to modifying communication strategies as the needs and abilities of the person with dementia change over time.

Effective communication in dementia care requires patience, empathy, and a willingness to adapt to the individual's unique needs and abilities. By employing these strategies, caregivers and family members can maintain meaningful connections and enhance the well-being of individuals living with dementia. Regular communication with healthcare professionals and experts in dementia care can offer additional guidance and insights into effective communication strategies.

Chapter 8

Connecting Through Memory and Reminiscence

Memory and reminiscence activities can be powerful tools for connecting with individuals living with dementia. These activities provide an opportunity to tap into the person's past experiences, evoke emotions, and foster meaningful interactions. One effective approach is using memory aids and memory books to engage individuals with dementia. Here's a detailed look at how these tools can be used:

1. Memory Aids:
Memory aids are physical or visual cues that help individuals with dementia recall memories, facts, or personal information. These aids can stimulate reminiscence, facilitate communication, and provide a sense of comfort. Some common memory aids include:

* Photographs: Family photos, pictures of past events, and snapshots from different life stages can trigger memories and stories. Display these photos or create a photo album for the person to view.

* Music: Music is a powerful memory trigger. Play songs from the person's youth or favorite music and encourage them to sing along or share their thoughts and feelings associated with the songs.

* Personal Items: Familiar objects, such as jewelry, clothing, or mementos, can bring back memories and serve as conversation starters.

* Scents and Fragrances: Certain scents, like perfumes or foods, can evoke memories. Using scented objects or products can help individuals reminisce about the past.

2. Memory Books:
Memory books, also known as life story books or reminiscence books, are collections of photos, documents, and written narratives that capture a person's life journey. These books offer a structured way to engage individuals with dementia in

reminiscence activities. Here's how to create and use memory books effectively:

* Collect Photos and Documents: Gather photographs, documents, and other memorabilia from different stages of the person's life, including childhood, young adulthood, marriage, and family life.

* Organize the Content: Arrange the collected items chronologically or thematically. Create sections or chapters within the memory book to represent different life periods or events.

* Include Descriptions: Write brief descriptions or narratives to accompany the photos and documents. Explain the significance of each item, such as who is in the photo or what the event was.

* Share and Discuss: Sit down with the person with dementia and explore the memory book together. Encourage them to look at the photos, read the descriptions, and share their memories and stories.

* Promote Conversation: Use open-ended questions to prompt discussions. For instance, "Tell me about

this picture" and "What do you remember from this time in your life?"

* Respect Emotions: Be prepared for a range of emotions that may arise during reminiscence. Some memories may evoke happiness, while others might bring sadness. Offer emotional support and understanding.

* Personalize the Book: Tailor the memory book to the individual's preferences and interests. Include items that are most meaningful to them.

* Keep the Book Accessible: Place the memory book in a location that is easily accessible to the person with dementia, such as their bedroom or a common area in the home.

* Regularly Update: As new memories are created, add them to the memory book to keep it current and reflective of the person's life.

Memory aids and memory books are valuable tools for promoting connection, communication, and emotional well-being in dementia care. They allow individuals to revisit their life stories and experiences, reinforcing their sense of identity and preserving a connection with their past. These reminiscence activities not only offer therapeutic benefits but also create meaningful opportunities for caregivers and family members to engage with and understand their loved ones on a deeper level.

Creating a Connection in Dementia Care

Creating a meaningful connection with individuals living with dementia is essential for their emotional well-being and quality of life. As cognitive abilities decline, maintaining a strong connection can become a more significant challenge, but it is also increasingly important. Here are strategies for creating and sustaining a connection in dementia care:

1. Be Present:
* Focused Attention: When interacting with the person with dementia, give them your full and undivided attention. Distractions like phones and other gadgets should be put aside.

* Non-Verbal Cues: Use non-verbal cues, such as eye contact, facial expressions, and body language, to convey warmth, empathy, and understanding.

2. Empathy and Understanding:
* Put Yourself in Their Shoes: Try to understand the person's emotions, frustrations, and needs from their perspective. This empathy can help you better relate to their experiences.

* Active Listening: Be an active listener. Pay close attention to both verbal and non-verbal cues to understand their feelings and thoughts.

3. Consistency and Routine:
* Predictable Schedule: Establish a predictable daily routine and consistent schedule for activities and mealtimes. Predictability can reduce anxiety and confusion.

* Familiar Environment: Keep the physical environment consistent to avoid disorientation. Avoid frequent changes to the home or living space.

4. Respect and Dignity:

*   Maintain Respect: Always treat the person with dementia with respect and dignity. Avoid speaking to them in a condescending or infantilizing manner.

*   Acknowledgment: Acknowledge their feelings, experiences, and preferences. Even if they can't express themselves fully, let them know that you value their input.

5. Share Memories:
*   Reminiscence: Use memory aids, memory books, or family photos to prompt reminiscence and discussions about their past experiences and memories.

*   Personal Stories: Share your own stories and experiences with the person. These shared moments can strengthen your bond and provide topics for conversation.

6. Physical Touch:
*   Comforting Gestures: Physical touch, such as holding hands or giving a comforting hug, can convey care and support. Ensure the person is comfortable with physical contact.

7. Be Patient:
* Flexibility: Recognize that the person with dementia may require more time to process information and respond. Avoid rushing them or showing frustration if they struggle to communicate.

* Repeat and Confirm: When necessary, repeat information and confirm to ensure mutual understanding. Be patient and adaptable in your interactions.

8. Promote Independence:
* Encourage Self-Care: Support the person in maintaining as much independence as possible in daily tasks, which can boost their self-esteem.

* Adapt and Simplify Tasks: Modify tasks as needed to make them more manageable, breaking them down into simpler steps if necessary.

9. Maintain Emotional Well-Being:
* Emotional Expression: Encourage the person to express their emotions, whether it's joy, frustration, or sadness. Validate their feelings and provide reassurance.

* Emotional Engagement: Engage in activities that evoke positive emotions, such as listening to music, engaging in art, or spending time in nature.

10. Seek Professional Support:
* Consult Experts: Don't hesitate to seek guidance from healthcare professionals and specialists in dementia care. They can offer insights and strategies tailored to the individual's needs.

Creating a connection in dementia care is a dynamic process that requires patience, empathy, and adaptability. It involves fostering a sense of trust, security, and understanding, even in the face of cognitive decline. By implementing these strategies, caregivers and family members can create and maintain a strong emotional connection that enhances the overall well-being and quality of life for individuals with dementia.

Chapter 9

Managing Challenging Behaviors in Dementia Care

Caring for individuals with dementia often involves addressing challenging behaviors that can arise as a result of the cognitive and neurological changes associated with the condition. Understanding the underlying causes and triggers of these behaviors is crucial for effective management and providing the best possible care. Here is an in-depth exploration of the understanding of challenging behaviors in dementia care:

1. Common Challenging Behaviors:

Understanding the types of challenging behaviors that can occur in dementia is a crucial first step. Some common challenging behaviors include:

¶ Agitation and Aggression: This can manifest as verbal or physical aggression, restlessness, or irritability.

¶ Wandering: Individuals with dementia may wander aimlessly, which can pose safety risks.

¶ Sundowning: Some people with dementia experience increased confusion and agitation in the late afternoon or evening.

¶ Hallucinations and Delusions: They may see or hear things that aren't there or hold false beliefs.

¶ Repetitive Behaviors: This can include repeatedly asking the same question or performing the same action.

¶ Inappropriate Social Behavior: This may involve making inappropriate comments, undressing in public, or acting impulsively.

¶ Resistance to Care: Individuals may resist help with personal care activities like bathing or dressing.

2. Causes of Challenging Behaviors:

Understanding the root causes of these behaviors is essential for effective management. Common causes include:

¶ Communication Difficulties: Many challenging behaviors arise from difficulty expressing needs or confusion. For example, aggression may result from frustration when the person can't communicate their discomfort.

¶ Physical Discomfort: Pain, illness, or discomfort can lead to agitation and other challenging behaviors.

¶ Environmental Factors: Changes in the environment, such as noise, overcrowding, or unfamiliar settings, can be distressing.

¶ Unmet Needs: The person may have unmet physical or emotional needs, such as hunger, thirst, or the need for social interaction.

¶ Medication Side Effects: Some medications can cause behavioral changes. It's important to monitor and adjust medications as needed.

¶ Past Trauma or Stress: Past traumatic experiences can influence behavior, especially in individuals with dementia.

3. Person-Centered Approach:

To effectively manage challenging behaviors, it's essential to adopt a person-centered approach, which recognizes that each individual is unique. This approach involves:

¶ Individualized Care: Tailoring care strategies to the person's specific needs and preferences.

¶ Respect and Dignity: Respecting the individual's dignity and autonomy at all times.

¶ Effective Communication: Using clear and empathetic communication to understand and address the person's needs.

4. Strategies for Managing Challenging Behaviors:

Based on the understanding of the causes, caregivers can employ various strategies to manage challenging behaviors:

¶ Communication: Use simple, clear language, and listen actively to understand the person's needs. Validate their feelings and reassure them.

¶ Prevent Triggers: Identify and minimize triggers in the environment. Create a calm and familiar setting.

¶ Structured Routine: Establish a daily routine to provide predictability and reduce anxiety.

¶ Redirect and Distract: When the person exhibits challenging behavior, redirect their attention to a different, more positive activity.

¶ Medication: In some cases, medications may be prescribed to manage severe challenging behaviors. Consult a healthcare professional for guidance.

¶ Calm and Reassure: Use a calm and reassuring approach to defuse agitation and distress.

¶ Offer Choices: Provide choices when appropriate to give the person a sense of control and autonomy.

¶ Professional Help: Seek assistance from healthcare professionals, including geriatric specialists or behavioral therapists, for more complex or persistent behaviors.

5. Safety Considerations:

Ensure the safety of the person with dementia and those around them. For example, if the person is prone to wandering, implement safety measures to prevent them from wandering into dangerous situations.

Understanding challenging behaviors in dementia care is a critical foundation for effective management. By identifying the causes, employing person-centered strategies, and focusing on the well-being of the individual, caregivers and healthcare professionals can provide the best possible care and improve the quality of life for individuals with dementia.

Agitation and Aggression in Dementia Care

Agitation and aggression are challenging behaviors that can manifest in individuals with dementia. These behaviors can be distressing for both the person with dementia and their caregivers. Understanding the underlying causes and implementing appropriate strategies is essential for managing and minimizing these behaviors in dementia care.

Understanding Agitation and Aggression:

¶ Agitation: Agitation refers to a state of restlessness, anxiety, and heightened activity. It can manifest as pacing, fidgeting, and a general sense of unease. Agitation in dementia is often a response to distress or an inability to communicate effectively. Common triggers for agitation include pain, discomfort, hunger, thirst, fear, confusion, or overstimulation.

¶ Aggression: Aggression involves physical or verbal behaviors that are meant to harm or intimidate. These behaviors may include hitting, pushing, yelling, or making threats. Aggression can be triggered by similar factors as agitation, such as physical discomfort, frustration, or a sense of threat.

Causes of Agitation and Aggression in Dementia

Understanding the root causes of these behaviors is essential for appropriate management. Common causes include:

¶ Pain and Discomfort: Individuals with dementia may be unable to express physical pain or discomfort verbally, leading to agitation or aggression.

¶ Communication Difficulties: The person may struggle to communicate their needs or frustrations, leading to agitation.

¶ Environmental Factors: Changes in the environment, such as excessive noise, unfamiliar settings, or overcrowding, can cause distress and agitation.

¶ Unmet Needs: Basic needs like hunger, thirst, or the need for social interaction may go unaddressed, leading to agitation.

¶ Fear and Anxiety: The person may experience fear or anxiety due to confusion, unfamiliar situations, or past traumatic experiences.

¶ Medication Side Effects: Some medications prescribed for dementia can lead to behavioral changes, including agitation and aggression.

Strategies for Managing Agitation and Aggression:

Managing agitation and aggression requires a multi-faceted approach that addresses the underlying causes and minimizes triggers. Here are some strategies to consider:

¶ Identify Triggers: Observe the person to identify specific triggers for their agitation or aggression. This can help you proactively address those triggers.

¶ Communication: Use simple and clear language when communicating with the person. Listen actively to their expressions and respond with empathy.

¶ Create a Calm Environment: Minimize environmental stressors by providing a calm and familiar setting. Reduce noise and clutter, and maintain a structured routine.

¶ Structured Routine: Establish a daily routine to provide predictability and reduce anxiety. Consistency can help the person feel more secure.

¶ Physical Comfort: Ensure the person is comfortable by addressing any physical discomfort, such as pain, hunger, or thirst.

¶ Medication Review: Consult a healthcare professional to review and adjust medications if they are contributing to the behavior.

¶ Redirection: When the person exhibits agitation or aggression, redirect their attention to a different, more positive activity or topic.

¶ Validation and Reassurance: Use a calm and reassuring approach to defuse agitation. Acknowledge their feelings and offer reassurance.

¶ Offer Choices: Provide choices whenever possible to give the person a sense of control and autonomy.

¶ Consult Professionals: Seek assistance from healthcare professionals, including geriatric specialists or behavioral therapists, for guidance on managing challenging behaviors.

¶ Safety Measures: Implement safety measures to prevent harm to the person or others in situations involving aggression.

Agitation and aggression in dementia care are complex and multifaceted challenges. Caregivers and healthcare professionals should work together to understand the specific triggers and underlying causes for each individual, develop personalized strategies, and provide a supportive and safe environment that promotes the person's overall well-being.

Sundowning in Dementia Care

Sundowning, also known as "sundown syndrome," is a common and challenging phenomenon that occurs in individuals with dementia. It's characterized by increased agitation, confusion, and behavioral changes in the late afternoon or evening, often continuing into the night. Understanding and managing sundowning is crucial for providing effective care to individuals with dementia.

Key Characteristics of Sundowning:

* Agitation: Individuals with sundowning may become more agitated, restless, and anxious as the day progresses, especially during the late afternoon and evening.

* Confusion: Sunsets frequently cause people to become more confused and disoriented. The person may not recognize familiar surroundings, objects, or even people.

* Irritability: Increased irritability and mood swings are common during sundowning episodes. The person may become easily frustrated or upset.

* Wandering: Some individuals with dementia may engage in wandering behavior during sundowning, which can pose safety risks.

* Sleep Disturbances: Sundowning can disrupt sleep patterns, leading to difficulty falling asleep and staying asleep throughout the night.

Causes of Sundowning:

The exact causes of sundowning are not fully understood, but several factors are believed to contribute to this phenomenon:

* Circadian Rhythm Disruption: Changes in the internal body clock can disrupt sleep-wake patterns, leading to increased confusion and agitation during the late afternoon and evening.

* Fatigue: Individuals with dementia may experience fatigue or "sundowning fatigue" as the

day progresses, which can exacerbate confusion and irritability.

* Low Lighting Levels: Reduced lighting in the evening can make it more difficult for individuals with dementia to perceive their surroundings accurately.

* Environmental Factors: Noise, unfamiliar surroundings, and other environmental factors can be more noticeable and distressing during the evening hours.

* Physical Discomfort: Physical discomfort, such as pain, hunger, or needing to use the restroom, can contribute to agitation during the late afternoon and evening.

Strategies for Managing Sundowning:

To manage sundowning effectively, caregivers can employ various strategies to minimize its impact and ensure the well-being of individuals with dementia:

* Establish a Routine: Maintain a consistent daily routine with set meal times, activities, and bedtime to provide predictability.

* Limit Stimulants: Reduce caffeine and sugar intake, especially in the afternoon and evening, to avoid exacerbating agitation.

* Increase Lighting: Ensure proper lighting in the evening to reduce confusion and improve the person's perception of their surroundings.

* Limit Napping: Discourage excessive daytime napping to help individuals feel more tired at night.

* Monitor Medications: Review the person's medications with a healthcare professional to identify any drugs that may be contributing to sundowning and consider adjusting the timing of medications.

* Engage in Calming Activities: Offer calming and enjoyable activities during the late afternoon and evening, such as listening to soothing music, reading, or engaging in gentle exercises.

* Provide a Relaxing Environment: Create a calm and quiet evening environment with minimal distractions and noise.

* Emphasize Sleep Hygiene: Promote good sleep hygiene practices, such as maintaining a comfortable sleep environment and avoiding stimulating activities close to bedtime.

* Consult Professionals: Seek advice from healthcare professionals and dementia care specialists for further guidance and strategies to manage sundowning.

Managing sundowning in dementia care requires a holistic approach that addresses environmental, physical, and psychological factors. By understanding the causes and employing appropriate strategies, caregivers can help individuals with dementia experience more peaceful and restful evenings while maintaining their overall well-being.

Chapter 10

Strategies for Dealing with Difficult Behaviors in Dementia Care

Caring for individuals with dementia often involves addressing difficult or challenging behaviors that can be distressing for both the person with dementia and their caregivers. These behaviors may include aggression, agitation, wandering, and resistance to care. Effective strategies for dealing with difficult behaviors are essential to provide the best possible care and ensure the well-being of individuals with dementia. Here is an in-depth discussion of these strategies:

1. Understand the Underlying Causes:
* Identify Triggers: Caregivers should observe and identify the specific triggers that lead to difficult behaviors. Common triggers include pain, discomfort, frustration, unmet needs, communication difficulties, environmental factors, and past trauma.

2. Person-Centered Care:
* Individualized Approach: Tailor care strategies to the person's specific needs, preferences, and history. Recognize that each individual is unique, and their care plan should reflect this.

* Respect and Dignity: Always treat the person with dementia with respect and dignity, maintaining their autonomy to the extent possible.

3. Effective Communication:
* Clear and Simple Language: Use simple and clear language when communicating with the person. Speak slowly and calmly, and give them time to respond.

* Active Listening: Pay close attention to both verbal and non-verbal cues to understand the person's feelings and thoughts.

* Validation: Acknowledge the person's feelings and experiences, even if they cannot express themselves fully. Validation can help reduce frustration and anxiety.

4. Prevent and Minimize Triggers:

* Create a Calm Environment: Minimize environmental stressors by providing a calm and familiar setting. Reduce the amount of noise, clutter, and confusion in the environment.

* Structured Routine: Establish a daily routine to provide predictability and reduce anxiety. Consistency can help the person feel more secure.

5. Safety Measures:
* Ensure Safety: Take steps to ensure the safety of the person with dementia and those around them, particularly in situations involving aggression or wandering.

* Wandering Prevention: Implement safety measures to prevent wandering, such as locking doors or using alarms.

6. Medication Management:
* Medication Review: Consult a healthcare professional to review and adjust medications if they are contributing to challenging behaviors.

7. Positive Reinforcement:

* Reward Positive Behavior: Use positive reinforcement to encourage and reward positive or desired behaviors. Praise and acknowledge the person when they exhibit behavior that is safe and appropriate.

8. Redirection and Distraction:
* Redirect Attention: When the person exhibits challenging behaviors, redirect their attention to a different, more positive activity or topic.

9. Professional Help:
* Consult Specialists: Seek assistance from healthcare professionals, including geriatric specialists or behavioral therapists, for more complex or persistent challenging behaviors.

10. Patience and Flexibility:
* Be Patient: Understand that dealing with difficult behaviors can be challenging, but it's essential to maintain patience and a calm demeanor.

* Adapt and Modify: Be adaptable and open to modifying care strategies as the needs and abilities of the person with dementia change over time.

11. Family and Caregiver Collaboration:
* Consistency: Ensure that all family members and caregivers use consistent approaches to dealing with difficult behaviors to avoid confusion and frustration for the individual with dementia.

Dealing with difficult behaviors in dementia care is a dynamic process that requires ongoing observation, patience, empathy, and adaptability. By implementing these strategies, caregivers and healthcare professionals can create a supportive and safe environment that promotes the well-being of individuals with dementia and enhances their overall quality of life.

Redirection and Distraction in Dementia Care

Redirection and distraction are valuable techniques in dementia care for managing challenging behaviors and diffusing potentially stressful or agitating situations. These strategies can be particularly effective when dealing with individuals with dementia who may exhibit behaviors such as aggression, agitation, repetitive actions, or anxiety.

Here's an in-depth look at redirection and distraction and how they can be used effectively:

1. Redirection:

Redirection involves shifting the person's focus or attention from a challenging or upsetting situation to a more positive and engaging one. The goal is to redirect their thoughts and feelings, thereby defusing tension and promoting a more pleasant interaction. Here's how redirection works:

* Identify Triggers: Recognize the specific triggers that lead to challenging behaviors. These triggers may be environmental, such as a noisy or crowded setting, or emotional, such as frustration or fear.

* Offer an Alternative Activity: When you notice the person becoming agitated or upset, gently introduce an alternative activity or topic of conversation that is likely to capture their interest.

* Use Positive Reinforcement: Praise the person for engaging in the redirected activity and provide positive reinforcement. This encourages them to continue with the new focus.

* Be Attentive: Pay close attention to the person's cues and responses. If the redirection isn't effective, be prepared to try a different approach or activity.

2. Distraction:

Distraction is a technique that involves diverting the person's attention away from a challenging situation or behavior by introducing a different stimulus or activity. Distraction aims to shift the person's focus so that they become less fixated on the challenging behavior. Here's how distraction works:

* Introduce a New Focus: When you notice the person engaging in a challenging behavior or becoming upset, introduce a new focus, such as offering them an interesting object or suggesting a pleasant activity.

* Use Sensory Stimuli: Sensory distractions can be effective, such as providing objects with different textures, colors, or scents. These can capture the person's attention and curiosity.

* Engage in Pleasant Activities: Suggest enjoyable activities that the person likes, such as listening to music, looking at family photos, or engaging in light physical exercises.

* Safety Considerations: Ensure that the distraction is safe and appropriate for the individual's cognitive and physical abilities.

3. Tips for Effective Redirection and Distraction:

* Know the Person: Understand the person's interests, preferences, and history. Tailor your redirection and distraction techniques to what you know will engage them.

* Stay Calm and Patient: Approach the person with a calm and patient demeanor. Avoid displaying frustration or impatience.

* Observe and Adapt: Continuously observe the person's reactions and adjust your approach as needed. What is effective one day may not be effective the next.

* Avoid Confrontation: Do not confront or argue with the person during challenging situations. This is unlikely to be productive and may escalate the behavior.

* Safety First: Ensure that the redirection and distraction techniques are safe and do not pose any harm to the person or others.

* Positive Reinforcement: Offer praise and positive reinforcement when the person successfully engages in the redirected or distracting activity.

Redirection and distraction are essential tools in dementia care for diffusing challenging behaviors and creating a more positive and comfortable environment for individuals with dementia. When used with sensitivity and creativity, these techniques can help both the person with dementia and their caregivers navigate challenging situations with less stress and more ease.

Calming Techniques in Dementia Care

Calming techniques are vital in dementia care to help individuals with dementia manage anxiety, agitation, and distress. These techniques aim to create a soothing and reassuring environment, reducing the potential for challenging behaviors and promoting overall well-being. Here is an overview of effective calming techniques for dementia care:

1. Create a Calm Environment:

* Reduce Noise: Minimize excessive noise and distractions in the living environment to create a quiet, calming atmosphere.

* Uncluttered Space: Keep living spaces neat and organized, as clutter can be overwhelming for individuals with dementia.

* Comfortable Lighting: Ensure that lighting is adequate and comfortable, especially in the evening to reduce confusion during sundowning.

* Familiarity: Surround the person with familiar objects, photos, and mementos that evoke positive memories and feelings of security.

2. Music Therapy:

* Music can have a profound calming effect: Play soothing and familiar music to help relax the individual. Music can evoke memories and improve mood.

* Personalized Playlists: Create a personalized playlist with the individual's favorite songs or music from their youth to make it more meaningful.

3. Gentle Physical Activities:

* Soothing Exercises: Encourage gentle physical activities like stretching, yoga, or tai chi to promote relaxation and reduce restlessness.

* Relaxation Techniques: Introduce relaxation techniques such as deep breathing exercises or meditation to help calm the person's mind.

4. Sensory Stimulation:

* Sensory Objects: Provide sensory items like stress balls, fidget toys, or textured objects that the person can touch and manipulate for comfort.

* Aromatherapy: Some individuals find relief in aromatherapy using calming scents like lavender, chamomile, or citrus. Be sure to consider any allergies or sensitivities.

5. Hand Massage and Touch:

* Hand massage: Gently massaging the person's hands can be soothing and provide a sense of comfort.

* Holding Hands: Holding the person's hand or offering a comforting touch can be reassuring.

6. Pet Therapy:

* Interacting with Pets: For individuals who enjoy animals, pet therapy or visits from therapy animals can have a calming and comforting effect.

7. Validation and Reassurance:

* Validation: Acknowledge the person's feelings and experiences, even if they cannot express

themselves fully. Validating their emotions can provide comfort.

* Reassurance: Offer words of reassurance and comfort, reminding the person that they are safe and cared for.

8. Diversion and Engagement:

* Diversion Activities: Engage the person in activities that capture their attention, such as looking at photo albums, reading, or completing simple puzzles.

* Structured Routine: Maintain a structured daily routine to provide predictability and reduce anxiety.

9. Provide Comfort Items:

* Comfort Objects: Offer comforting items like blankets, stuffed animals, or favorite possessions that provide a sense of security.

10. Be Attentive and Patient:

* Observation: Pay close attention to the person's cues and reactions, and adapt your approach as needed. What is effective one day may not be effective the next.

* Patience: Approach the person with patience, empathy, and understanding. Avoid displaying frustration or impatience.

11. Professional Guidance:

* Consult Specialists: Seek advice from healthcare professionals, including dementia specialists, who can provide tailored strategies for calming techniques based on the individual's unique needs.

Using calming techniques in dementia care helps reduce anxiety and improve the quality of life for individuals living with dementia. These techniques create a supportive and nurturing environment that promotes a sense of well-being, security, and comfort, fostering positive interactions and reducing the likelihood of challenging behaviors.

Chapter 11

Seeking Professional Help in Dementia Care

Caring for a loved one with dementia can be emotionally and physically demanding. While many caregivers provide care at home, there may come a time when professional assistance becomes necessary to ensure the well-being and safety of the individual with dementia and to support the primary caregiver. Knowing when to consider professional care is essential for providing the best care possible. Here are some indicators of when to seek professional help in dementia care:

1. Progressive Decline in Cognitive Abilities:
As dementia progresses, the care needs become more complex. If the individual's cognitive decline reaches a point where it's challenging for the primary caregiver to manage, it's time to consider professional care.

2. Safety Concerns:

If the person with dementia exhibits behaviors that pose a risk to their safety or the safety of others, such as wandering, aggression, or falls, it's important to seek professional care to address these safety concerns.

3. Caregiver Burnout:

Caregiver burnout is a significant concern in dementia care. When the primary caregiver feels overwhelmed, stressed, or physically exhausted, it may be time to consider professional help to provide respite and support.

4. Lack of Necessary Skills:

Providing care for someone with advanced dementia requires specific skills and knowledge. If the primary caregiver lacks these skills or is struggling to meet the individual's care needs, professional assistance is essential.

5. Medical and Health Needs:

As dementia progresses, individuals may develop other health conditions that require medical attention. Professional caregivers can provide the necessary medical and healthcare support.

6. Behavioral and Psychological Symptoms:
The presence of challenging behaviors, such as severe agitation, aggression, hallucinations, or delusions, may necessitate the involvement of professionals who specialize in managing these symptoms.

7. Personal Hygiene and Care:
When the person with dementia is unable to manage personal hygiene, dressing, or toileting independently, professional caregivers can assist with these activities of daily living.

8. Social Isolation:
Dementia caregivers often face social isolation as they become increasingly focused on the care recipient. Seeking professional care can help alleviate this isolation and provide opportunities for social engagement and support.

9. Medication Management:
As individuals with dementia may require multiple medications, managing medication schedules, doses, and potential side effects can become complex. Professional assistance can ensure proper medication management.

10. Respite and Support:
Caregivers need respite to rest and recharge. Professional care services, such as adult day care or in-home respite care, provide caregivers with the support they need.

11. Legal and Financial Planning:
If there are concerns about financial exploitation, legal issues, or difficulties managing finances, seeking professional help, such as a financial advisor or attorney, is crucial.

12. Hospice and End-of-Life Care:
In the advanced stages of dementia, when end-of-life care is needed, professional hospice care services can provide comfort, pain management, and emotional support for both the individual and their family.

13. Consult with Healthcare Professionals:
Consult with healthcare professionals, including geriatric specialists, neurologists, or dementia experts, for guidance on when to transition to professional care.

14. Family Decision:
Deciding to seek professional care is a family decision. It's important to involve family members in the decision-making process and consider the input and preferences of the person with dementia when possible.

Transitioning to professional care in dementia can be challenging, but it's often a necessary step to ensure the safety, well-being, and quality of life of the individual with dementia and the primary caregiver. Seek advice and support from healthcare professionals, support organizations, and care providers to navigate this transition effectively.

In-Home Care in Dementia Care

In-home care is a popular choice for many families caring for a loved one with dementia. It allows the individual to remain in their familiar environment while receiving professional assistance. In-home care services can vary widely, and they can be adapted to meet the specific needs and preferences of the individual with dementia and their family.

Here's an in-depth look at in-home care in dementia care:

1. Types of In-Home Care:

° Companion Care: Companion caregivers provide social interaction, emotional support, and assistance with light household tasks. They help reduce loneliness and offer companionship.

° Personal Care Assistants (PCAs): PCAs assist with activities of daily living (ADLs) such as bathing, dressing, grooming, and toileting. They may also provide assistance with mobility.

° Home Health Care: Home health care services include medical care provided by licensed healthcare professionals. It can involve medication management, wound care, and monitoring of health conditions.

° Respite Care: Respite care is temporary care that allows the primary caregiver to take a break. This type of care can be beneficial for preventing caregiver burnout.

° Hospice Care: In-home hospice care focuses on providing comfort and support to individuals in the advanced stages of dementia at the end of life.

2. Benefits of In-Home Care:

° Familiar Environment: In-home care allows the person with dementia to remain in a familiar and comfortable environment, reducing confusion and anxiety.

° Personalized Care: In-home care services can be tailored to the individual's specific needs and preferences, providing a more personalized approach to care.

° Family Involvement: In-home care often encourages family involvement and participation in the care process, which can be comforting for the individual and their loved ones.

° Consistency: The individual can maintain a consistent daily routine, which can be soothing and reduce anxiety.

3. Services Offered:

○ Assistance with Activities of Daily Living (ADLs): In-home caregivers can help with bathing, dressing, grooming, toileting, and other personal care tasks.

○ Medication Management: Caregivers can assist with medication reminders and administration.

○ Meal Preparation: They can help plan and prepare meals, ensuring the person with dementia receives proper nutrition.

○ Household Tasks: Caregivers can assist with light housekeeping, laundry, and other household chores.

○ Companionship: Providing companionship, conversation, and social engagement to reduce feelings of isolation and loneliness.

○ Mobility Assistance: Helping the person move safely to prevent falls or accidents.

○ Transportation: Assisting with transportation to medical appointments, social outings, or other activities.

° Safety Supervision: Ensuring the individual's safety by monitoring them and addressing any immediate safety concerns.

4. Cost of In-Home Care:

The cost of in-home care can vary widely based on the type and amount of care required, the geographic location, and the qualifications of the caregivers. Some individuals may be eligible for financial assistance or government programs to help cover the cost.

5. Caregiver Training:

It's essential to ensure that in-home caregivers are well-trained in dementia care, including understanding the specific needs and behaviors associated with dementia. They should also have experience and skills in dealing with challenging behaviors and communication strategies.

6. Ongoing Assessment:

Regular assessments of the individual's care needs should be conducted, and the care plan should be adjusted as the dementia progresses or changes occur in the person's condition.

In-home care provides a viable option for families seeking to support a loved one with dementia while allowing them to remain in their home. It offers a range of services that can be tailored to the individual's unique needs, providing comfort, consistency, and personalized care. Families should carefully evaluate their options, seek recommendations, and choose an in-home care provider that specializes in dementia care.

Assisted Living and Memory Care Facilities in Dementia Care

Assisted living and memory care facilities are residential options that cater to individuals with dementia who need various levels of support and care. These facilities are designed to provide a safe, supportive, and engaging environment for people living with dementia. Here's an in-depth discussion of assisted living and memory care facilities in dementia care:

1. Assisted Living Facilities:

• General Support: Assisted living facilities are designed to provide a supportive and communal environment for seniors who need assistance with daily activities but do not require round-the-clock medical care.

• Dementia-Friendly: Many assisted living facilities have separate units or areas dedicated to dementia care. These units are staffed by caregivers with specialized training in dementia care.

• Services: Residents in assisted living facilities receive assistance with tasks like bathing, dressing, medication management, meal preparation, and housekeeping.

• Social Engagement: Assisted living facilities often offer a variety of social and recreational activities to keep residents engaged and stimulated.

• Independence: Residents typically have a degree of independence and can participate in decision-making regarding their care.

• Transition to Memory Care: If the individual's dementia progresses to a point where they require more specialized care and supervision, they can transition to a dedicated memory care unit within the facility.

2. Memory Care Facilities:

• Specialized Dementia Care: Memory care facilities are specifically designed to cater to the unique needs of individuals with dementia, particularly those with moderate to severe symptoms.

• Secure Environment: These facilities often have secure entry and exit points to prevent wandering and ensure the safety of residents.

• Trained Staff: Caregivers in memory care facilities receive specialized training in dementia care and are skilled in dealing with challenging behaviors.

• Activities and Therapies: Memory care facilities offer a range of activities and therapies tailored to stimulate cognitive functions and promote a sense of well-being.

• Structured Routine: A structured daily routine helps individuals with dementia maintain consistency, which can be calming and reduce anxiety.

• Personalized Care: Care plans are individualized to meet the unique needs of each resident, considering their abilities and preferences.

• Safety Measures: These facilities are equipped with safety features like handrails, non-slip flooring, and alarm systems to prevent accidents and injuries.

3. Cost of Care:

• The cost of assisted living and memory care facilities can vary based on factors such as the location, level of care required, and the facility's amenities. Memory care facilities, being more specialized and offering a higher level of care, are often more expensive than assisted living.

4. Family Involvement:

• Family members are encouraged to be involved in the care of their loved ones in both types of facilities. Many facilities offer family support and education programs to help family members understand and cope with the challenges of dementia care.

5. Choosing the Right Facility:

• When selecting an assisted living or memory care facility, it's important to consider factors such as the level of care needed, the facility's reputation, staff training, and the environment that would be most suitable for the individual with dementia.

• Visiting multiple facilities, speaking with staff, and seeking recommendations from other families who have experience with the facility can be helpful in making an informed choice.

Assisted living and memory care facilities offer specialized care and support for individuals with dementia, allowing them to live in a safe and engaging environment that is designed to meet their unique needs. Family involvement, along with a thoughtful evaluation of the individual's requirements and preferences, is crucial in selecting the right facility to provide the best quality of life for those living with dementia.

Chapter 12

Legal and Financial Considerations in Dementia Care

Caring for a loved one with dementia involves various legal and financial considerations. Navigating these aspects can be complex, but it's essential to ensure the person with dementia's well-being and protect their rights. Here's an in-depth discussion of legal and financial considerations in dementia care:

Legal Considerations:

1. Advance Directives:

* Advance Healthcare Directives: These documents, including a living will and healthcare power of attorney, allow the person with dementia to specify their medical wishes and designate someone to make healthcare decisions on their behalf.

* Power of Attorney: A durable power of attorney for finances designates someone to manage the person's financial affairs if they become unable to do so themselves.

2. Guardianship and Conservatorship:

* If the person with dementia has not appointed a power of attorney, and their cognitive decline prevents them from making informed decisions, a family member or legal guardian may need to seek guardianship or conservatorship to manage their affairs.

3. Estate Planning:

* Estate planning, including creating or updating a will, can help ensure that the person's assets and property are distributed according to their wishes.

4. Protection from Exploitation:

* Individuals with dementia are vulnerable to financial exploitation. Family members should be vigilant in monitoring financial transactions and protecting the person's assets.

5. Legal Capacity:

* If questions arise about the person's legal capacity to make decisions, a legal capacity assessment may be required to determine their ability to manage their personal and financial affairs.

Financial Considerations:

1. Care Costs:

* The cost of dementia care can be substantial, depending on the level of care needed. Consider factors like in-home care, assisted living, or memory care facilities, and their associated expenses.

2. Insurance:

* Long-term care insurance or Medicaid may help cover the costs of care. It's important to understand the terms of insurance policies and the eligibility criteria for Medicaid.

3. Financial Planning:

* Create a financial plan that outlines the person's assets, income, and projected expenses. This plan can help in managing funds and making informed decisions.

4. Public Benefits:

* Investigate whether the person is eligible for public benefits, such as Social Security, Supplemental Security Income (SSI), or Veterans Affairs (VA) benefits.

5. Asset Protection:

* Consider asset protection strategies, including trusts or gifting, to safeguard the person's assets while complying with legal requirements.

6. Professional Guidance:

* Seek advice from financial advisors, elder law attorneys, and geriatric care managers to develop a comprehensive financial plan and understand the options available.

7. Tax Considerations:

* Be aware of potential tax implications of financial decisions, and explore tax credits or deductions for healthcare expenses and caregiver support.

8. Document Management:

* Maintain thorough records of financial transactions, healthcare expenses, and legal documents for easy access and to facilitate communication with financial and legal professionals.

Family Communication:

• Open and honest communication among family members is crucial to ensure that everyone is aware of the legal and financial aspects of dementia care. Establish a clear plan for sharing responsibilities and making important decisions.

Navigating the legal and financial aspects of dementia care can be challenging, but it's essential to ensure the person's well-being and protect their rights. Engage professionals who specialize in elder law, financial planning, and dementia care to provide guidance and support in making informed decisions that best serve the person with dementia and their family.

Power of Attorney and Advance Directives in Dementia Care

Power of Attorney (POA) and Advance Directives are legal documents that play a crucial role in ensuring that the wishes and interests of individuals with dementia are upheld when they are no longer able to make decisions for themselves. Understanding these legal instruments is essential in dementia care:

What is a Power of Attorney (POA)?

A Power of Attorney is a legal document that gives one person (the principal) the ability to act on behalf of another (the agent or attorney-in-fact). This can include making financial, legal, and medical decisions.

Types of Power of Attorney:

¶ General Power of Attorney: Provides broad powers to the agent, but it is often revoked if the principal becomes incapacitated.

¶ Durable Power of Attorney: Continues to function in the event that the principal loses capacity. This is particularly important in dementia care to allow the agent to make decisions when the individual can no longer do so.

¶ Springing Power of Attorney: Becomes effective only when specific conditions, such as incapacity, are met.

How Power of Attorney Works in Dementia Care:

In dementia care, the individual with dementia appoints an agent to manage their financial and legal affairs. This agent can pay bills, manage investments, and make legal decisions when the person with dementia is no longer capable.

What are Advance Directives?

Advance Directives are legal documents that allow individuals to express their medical wishes and preferences in advance, especially concerning end-of-life care. Advance directives typically come in two forms:

¶ Living Will: A living will specifies the medical treatments the individual wishes to receive or avoid, particularly in life-threatening or end-of-life situations.

¶ Healthcare Power of Attorney: This document designates a healthcare proxy or agent to make medical decisions on the individual's behalf when they are unable to do so.

How Advance Directives Work in Dementia Care:

In dementia care, advance directives can be invaluable, as they specify the individual's preferences for medical care when they can no longer express their wishes. These documents guide healthcare providers and family members in making decisions that align with the person's values and desires.

Importance of POA and Advance Directives in Dementia Care:

- Dementia is a progressive condition, and as cognitive abilities decline, individuals may reach a point where they are no longer capable of making informed decisions. Having a durable power of attorney and advance directives in place ensures that:

- The person's financial, legal, and medical decisions are made by trusted individuals who are aware of their wishes.

- The individual's values and preferences regarding healthcare are respected, even if they cannot communicate them directly.

- Avoidance of conflicts among family members and healthcare providers regarding treatment decisions.

- A clear legal framework for making important decisions, which can alleviate stress for family members and caregivers.

Creating POA and Advance Directives:

To create Power of Attorney and Advance Directives, it is advisable to consult with an attorney who specializes in elder law or estate planning. The attorney can help draft the documents, ensure they comply with state laws, and answer any legal questions.

Regular Review:

It is essential to regularly review and update these documents, especially in the context of dementia care, as the individual's condition and preferences may change over time.
Ensuring that Power of Attorney and Advance Directives are established and executed in dementia care is vital for safeguarding the well-being and ensuring the individual's wishes are respected, even when they are no longer able to express them directly. Consulting with legal professionals who have expertise in elder law is recommended to navigate these complex legal matters.

Managing Finances and Insurance in Dementia Care

Caring for a loved one with dementia often involves complex financial and insurance considerations. Proper management of finances and insurance is crucial to ensure the well-being of the individual with dementia and to provide financial security for their future. Here is an in-depth discussion of managing finances and insurance in dementia care:

1. Financial Management:

* Create a Financial Plan: Develop a comprehensive financial plan that outlines the individual's assets, income, and projected expenses related to their care. This plan should provide a clear picture of the financial resources available for dementia care.

* Budgeting: Establish a budget that accounts for ongoing care expenses, such as in-home care, memory care facilities, medical costs, and support services.

* Legal and Financial Advisors: Consult with financial advisors and elder law attorneys who specialize in dementia care. They can offer guidance on managing assets, estate planning, and navigating complex financial matters.

* Monitoring and Record-Keeping: Maintain detailed records of financial transactions, healthcare expenses, and legal documents. Effective record-keeping helps in managing finances and ensures transparency.

* Medicaid and Public Benefits: Determine whether the individual is eligible for public benefits like Medicaid, which can help cover the costs of long-term care services. These programs often have income and asset limits, and eligibility requirements may vary by state.

2. Insurance Considerations:

* Long-Term Care Insurance: Long-term care insurance can be a valuable resource to cover the costs of dementia care. Review the terms and conditions of the policy and understand what types of care and services are covered.

* Health Insurance: Understand the individual's health insurance coverage, including Medicare and supplemental insurance. Know what medical

expenses are covered, including doctor visits, hospital stays, and prescription medications.

* Life Insurance: Some life insurance policies offer accelerated death benefits, which allow individuals to access a portion of their policy's death benefit to cover the costs of long-term care.

* Consideration of Annuities: Annuities can provide a regular income stream that may help cover the costs of dementia care. However, it's important to assess the terms and potential tax implications.

* Review Existing Policies: Review and understand the terms of all insurance policies, and consult with an insurance professional to explore options for enhancing coverage or addressing coverage gaps.

3. Protection from Exploitation:

* Preventing Financial Exploitation: Individuals with dementia are vulnerable to financial exploitation. It is essential to monitor financial transactions and protect the person's assets. Consider establishing safeguards to prevent unauthorized access to funds.

4. Tax Considerations:

* Be aware of potential tax implications of financial decisions, such as the tax treatment of insurance payouts or expenses related to dementia care. Explore tax credits or deductions for healthcare expenses and caregiver support.

5. Professional Guidance:

* Seek advice from financial advisors, insurance professionals, and legal experts who specialize in elder care and dementia. They can help navigate complex financial and insurance matters and provide tailored solutions.

6. Family Communication:

* Open and transparent communication among family members is vital to ensure that everyone is aware of the financial and insurance aspects of dementia care. Establish a clear plan for sharing responsibilities and making important financial decisions.

Effective management of finances and insurance is critical in dementia care to provide the best possible care while safeguarding the financial well-being of the individual with dementia. Seeking professional guidance and maintaining clear communication within the family can help navigate the complexities of managing finances and insurance in the context of dementia care.

Chapter 13

Self-Care for Caregivers

Caring for a loved one with dementia can be emotionally and physically demanding. To provide the best care possible, it's essential for caregivers to prioritize self-care. Here's an in-depth discussion of self-care for caregivers:

1. Understanding the Importance of Self-Care:

Self-care is not selfish; it's necessary for the well-being of both the caregiver and the person with dementia. When caregivers take care of themselves, they can provide better care to their loved one.

2. Recognizing Caregiver Stress and Burnout:

Caregiver stress and burnout are common in dementia care. Signs include fatigue, feelings of overwhelm, anxiety, depression, and physical ailments. The first step in treating these symptoms is identifying them.

3. Prioritizing Self-Care:

¶ Respite Care: Arrange for respite care so that you can take brief breaks from caregiving. This can involve family members, friends, or professional caregivers who can step in temporarily.

¶ Seek Support: Join caregiver support groups to connect with others who understand your challenges. Seek emotional support and share experiences.

¶ Delegate Tasks: Never be afraid to assign chores to friends or other family members. You do not have to do everything on your own.

¶ Set Realistic Expectations: Acknowledge your limitations and establish reasonable goals for your capabilities. Understand that you cannot control every aspect of the person's dementia.

¶ Maintain a Social Life: Continue engaging with your social circle. Isolation can contribute to caregiver stress, so make an effort to spend time with friends and family.

¶ Physical Health: Prioritize your physical health by eating well, staying active, and getting enough sleep. Good physical health is essential for managing caregiver stress.

¶ Psychological Well-being: Take up stress-relieving activities like yoga, meditation, or deep breathing. Seek counseling or therapy if you're experiencing persistent emotional distress.

¶ Regular Respite: Schedule regular respite time where you can engage in activities you enjoy. Whether it's reading, gardening, or hobbies, taking time for yourself is essential.

¶ Accept Help: Accept help when it is offered without hesitation. Often, friends and family are willing to assist if you communicate your needs.

¶ Consult with Professionals: Speak with healthcare professionals and social workers who can provide guidance and support tailored to your situation.

4. Strategies for Managing Stress:

¶ Time Management: Organize your schedule to manage caregiving tasks efficiently. Prioritize tasks and focus on the most critical needs.

¶ Communication: Communicate openly and honestly with your loved one's healthcare team. Ask questions, seek clarification, and express your concerns.

¶ Set Boundaries: Establish clear boundaries for your caregiving role. This includes setting limits on the time and energy you can dedicate to caregiving without neglecting your own needs.

¶ Acceptance: Accept that there will be difficult moments and that you may not have all the answers. Be kind to yourself and recognize that you're doing your best.

5. Resilience and Self-Compassion:

Building resilience and practicing self-compassion are vital in self-care. You're not expected to be perfect, and it's okay to ask for help and take care of yourself.

Caring for someone with dementia is a challenging and demanding role. However, caregivers should remember that taking care of themselves is not a sign of weakness but a necessity. Self-care is essential to maintain good physical and mental health, ensuring that caregivers can continue to provide quality care for their loved ones while also maintaining their own well-being.

Avoiding Burnout in Dementia Care

Caring for a loved one with dementia can be emotionally and physically exhausting, often leading to caregiver burnout. To provide effective care while maintaining your own well-being, it's crucial to recognize and take steps to avoid burnout. Here's an in-depth discussion on how to avoid burnout in dementia care:

`1. Recognizing the Signs of Burnout:

- Emotional Exhaustion: Feeling overwhelmed, irritable, or emotionally drained.

- Physical Fatigue: Experiencing physical symptoms like headaches, sleep disturbances, or weakened immunity.
- Reduced Personal Fulfillment: Feeling a sense of hopelessness, helplessness, or that your efforts are in vain.
- Neglecting Self-Care: Neglecting your own well-being, health, and interests to prioritize the care recipient's needs.
- Social Isolation: Withdrawing from friends and family, often due to the demands of caregiving.

2. Maintain a Balanced Perspective:

Remember that caregiving is just one aspect of your life. While it is a significant responsibility, it is essential to maintain balance by continuing to engage in personal and social activities.

3. Seek Professional Help:

If you notice persistent signs of burnout, such as anxiety or depression, it may be necessary to seek professional counseling or therapy to address these issues effectively.

4. Celebrate Small Achievements:

Recognize and celebrate the small achievements and moments of joy that occur in your caregiving journey. These moments can help provide a sense of purpose and fulfillment.

Avoiding burnout in dementia care is essential to ensure that you can provide the best care possible while maintaining your own physical and emotional well-being. Caregivers should understand that self-care is not a sign of weakness but a necessary component of sustaining their ability to provide effective and compassionate care for their loved ones.

Finding Support and Respite in Dementia Care

Caring for a loved one with dementia can be emotionally and physically challenging, making it crucial to find support and respite to maintain your own well-being as a caregiver. Here's an in-depth discussion on finding support and respite in dementia care:

1. Importance of Support and Respite:

- Support and respite are vital components of dementia care because they help caregivers to:
- Reduce caregiver stress and prevent burnout.
- Maintain physical and mental health.
- Improve the quality of care provided to the person with dementia.
- Avoid social isolation and seek emotional support.

2. Sources of Support:

¶ Caregiver Support Groups: Join local or online caregiver support groups. These provide a platform to connect with others facing similar challenges, share experiences, and receive valuable advice and support.

¶ Friends and Family: Share your caregiving responsibilities with trusted family members or friends. They can provide physical and emotional assistance.

¶ Professional Caregivers: Consider hiring professional caregivers or respite care services. These trained individuals can take over caregiving duties for short periods to allow you to take a break.

¶ Healthcare Professionals: Consult with healthcare providers and social workers who can guide you through the care process and connect you with appropriate resources.

¶ Alzheimer's Associations and Organizations: Organizations such as the Alzheimer's Association provide educational resources, support, and local chapter meetings.

¶ Support from Faith and Community Groups: Many faith-based and community organizations offer support for caregivers. This can include practical assistance, emotional support, and respite care.

3. Respite Care Options:

* In-Home Respite Care: Professional caregivers can come to your home to provide care while you take a break. They can help with daily tasks and companionship.

* Adult Day Care: Adult day care centers offer a safe and engaging environment for the person with dementia, allowing caregivers to work or take time for themselves during the day.

* Residential Respite Care: Some memory care facilities offer short-term residential respite care for individuals with dementia. This option can be helpful when a longer break is needed.

* Supportive Services: Many communities have supportive services, such as Meals on Wheels or transportation assistance, which can provide relief for caregivers.

4. Strategies to Access Support and Respite:

* Ask for Help: Don't be afraid to ask family members, friends, or support groups for assistance. People are often willing to help when they know your needs.

* Plan and Schedule Respite: Schedule regular respite breaks into your caregiving routine. This ensures you have dedicated time for self-care.

* Explore Local Resources: Research local support services, community organizations, and government programs that can provide support and respite.

* Use Technology: Consider using technology and online resources to connect with support groups and access virtual respite options.

* Financial Assistance: Explore financial assistance options to help cover the costs of professional respite care services.

* Self-Care During Respite: While taking respite, use the time for self-care activities, such as exercise, relaxation, or engaging in hobbies and interests.

6. Regular Communication: Maintain regular communication with those providing support or respite care to ensure a smooth transition and consistency in the care provided.

Finding support and respite in dementia care is crucial for both the caregiver's well-being and the quality of care provided to the person with dementia. Caregivers should reach out to various sources of support and regularly schedule respite time to prevent burnout and maintain their physical and emotional health.

Chapter 14

Planning for the Future in Dementia Care

Planning for the future when caring for a loved one with dementia is essential to ensure that the person with dementia receives the best care possible and that their legal, financial, and healthcare needs are met. Here's an in-depth discussion on planning for the future in dementia care:

1. Legal and Financial Planning:

i. Power of Attorney (POA): Appoint a durable power of attorney for both financial and healthcare decisions. This designates someone to make decisions when the person with dementia is no longer able to do so.

ii. Advance Directives: Create advance directives, including a living will and a healthcare power of attorney, to specify medical wishes and designate a healthcare proxy.

iii. Guardianship and Conservatorship: In cases where there is no POA or advance directives, it may be necessary to seek guardianship or conservatorship through the legal system to manage the person's affairs.

iv. Estate Planning: Engage in estate planning to ensure that the person's assets and property are distributed according to their wishes. This may include creating or updating a will, establishing trusts, and designating beneficiaries.

v. Asset Protection: Explore strategies to protect the person's assets, including trusts or gifting, while complying with legal requirements.

vi. Financial Management:Develop a comprehensive financial plan that outlines the individual's assets, income, and projected expenses related to their care. This helps in managing funds effectively.

2. Advance Care Planning:

Encourage the person with dementia to be actively involved in advance care planning, sharing their values and preferences with healthcare providers and family members.

* Health Records and Documentation:

Maintain a comprehensive record of the person's medical history, current medications, and healthcare documents. This information is essential for healthcare providers and family members.

3. Family Communication:

Engage in open and honest communication with family members to ensure that everyone is aware of the person's wishes and the plans for their care. Clearly define the roles and responsibilities of each family member.

4. Regular Reviews and Updates:

Regularly review and update legal documents, financial plans, and care preferences. The needs and wishes of the person with dementia may change over time.

5. Seek Professional Guidance:

Consult with professionals who specialize in elder law, financial planning, and dementia care to provide guidance and support in making informed decisions and navigating complex legal and financial matters.

Planning for the future in dementia care is crucial to ensure that the person with dementia receives the care they desire and that their legal, financial, and healthcare needs are met. Engaging in open communication, seeking professional advice, and regularly reviewing and updating plans are essential to adapt to changing circumstances and provide the best quality of care.

Long-Term Care Planning in Dementia Care

Long-term care planning is a critical component of providing comprehensive care for individuals with dementia. It involves making arrangements for the ongoing care and support of the person with dementia, addressing their medical, financial, and personal needs. Here's an in-depth discussion of long-term care planning in dementia care:

1. Determine Care Preferences:
Start by discussing and understanding the person with dementia's care preferences. This includes their desires related to where and how they wish to receive care. Consider their preferences for remaining at home, moving to an assisted living facility, or transitioning to a specialized memory care unit.

2. Long-Term Care Insurance:
Evaluate the benefits of long-term care insurance. This type of insurance is designed to cover the costs of extended care services. Review the policy terms, coverage options, and understand what types of care and services are included.

3. Medicaid and Public Benefits:
Determine if the person with dementia is eligible for Medicaid or other public benefits that can help cover the costs of long-term care services. Medicaid is a government program that provides assistance to individuals with limited income and assets.

4. Evaluate Care Settings:

• In-Home Care: Explore the possibility of in-home care, where professional caregivers provide support and assistance while allowing the person to remain in a familiar environment.

• Assisted Living: Assisted living facilities provide a level of care that allows individuals to maintain some independence while receiving support with daily activities.

• Memory Care Units: Memory care units are specialized facilities designed to cater specifically to individuals with dementia. They offer a skilled workforce in a controlled, safe setting.

• Hospice and Palliative Care: Consider options for hospice and palliative care as the disease progresses and the focus shifts toward providing comfort and symptom management.

5. Legal and Financial Planning:
Ensure that legal and financial plans are in place to support long-term care. This includes appointing a

durable power of attorney, creating advance directives, and addressing estate planning.

6. Advance Care Planning:

Engage in advance care planning discussions to clarify the person's medical wishes and preferences for end-of-life care. This includes decisions about resuscitation, artificial nutrition, and other medical interventions.

7. Document Care Preferences:

Document and share the person's care preferences and medical wishes with healthcare providers, family members, and caregivers. This ensures that everyone involved in the care process is aware of the person's desires.

8. Review and Update Plans:

Regularly review and update long-term care plans as the needs and wishes of the person with dementia may change over time. It's important to adapt the care plan to evolving circumstances.

9. Seek Professional Guidance:

Consult with professionals who specialize in elder law, financial planning, and dementia care to provide guidance and support in making informed decisions and navigating complex legal and financial matters.

10. Family Communication:
Maintain open and transparent communication with family members to ensure that everyone is on the same page regarding the long-term care plan. Clearly define the roles and responsibilities of each family member.

Long-term care planning is a comprehensive process that involves making decisions about the care and support of a person with dementia as the disease progresses. It's important to align the plan with the individual's care preferences, legal and financial arrangements, and regularly review and update the plan to ensure it remains responsive to their changing needs. Consulting with professionals and involving family members in the planning process is crucial to provide the best quality of care.

End-of-Life Care Decisions in Dementia Care

End-of-life care decisions are a sensitive and crucial aspect of dementia care, as the disease's progression eventually reaches a point where care focuses on comfort and quality of life. End-of-life care decisions in dementia care require careful consideration, open communication, and respect for the person's values and preferences. It's crucial to provide comfort, dignity, and support to both the individual with dementia and their family members during this challenging time. Consulting with healthcare professionals and legal experts is recommended to ensure that all decisions align with ethical and legal standards.

Chapter 15

Creating a Happy and Comfortable Life in Dementia Care: Activities and Engagement

Creating a happy and comfortable life for individuals with dementia is essential for their well-being and quality of life. Activities and engagement play a significant role in achieving this goal. Here's an in-depth discussion of activities and engagement in dementia care:

1. Importance of Activities and Engagement:

Engaging activities are vital for individuals with dementia as they provide a sense of purpose, reduce anxiety, and improve overall mood and well-being. Meaningful engagement also helps maintain cognitive and physical abilities for as long as possible.

2. Person-Centered Care: The foundation of successful activities and engagement in dementia care is person-centered care. This approach

recognizes the unique needs, preferences, and abilities of the individual with dementia.

3. Tailored Activities: Select activities that are tailored to the person's interests, hobbies, and past experiences. These activities are more likely to be engaging and enjoyable.

4. Cognitive and Sensory Stimulation

* Cognitive Activities: Engage the person in cognitive exercises such as puzzles, word games, or reminiscing about past experiences. These activities help maintain mental acuity and provide a sense of accomplishment.

* Sensory Stimulation: Activities that stimulate the senses, such as listening to music, smelling familiar scents, or feeling different textures, can provide comfort and enhance the sensory experience.

5. Physical Activities: Encourage light physical activities like walking, stretching, or chair exercises. Physical activity supports overall health, reduces restlessness, and promotes better sleep.

6. Creative Expression,: Activities that involve creative expression, such as painting, drawing, or crafting, allow individuals to express themselves and tap into their artistic abilities.

7. Social Interaction: Facilitate opportunities for social interaction. Group activities, family visits, and conversations help combat feelings of isolation and promote a sense of belonging.

8. Structured Routine: Establish a daily routine with consistent meal times, activities, and rest periods. Predictability can provide a sense of comfort and security.

9. Multi-Sensory Environments:
Create multi-sensory environments with various sensory experiences like soothing lights, music, and tactile elements to engage the individual's senses.

10. Memory Aids: Use memory aids like memory books or memory boxes to trigger reminiscence and foster a connection to the past.

11. Encourage Independence: Whenever possible, encourage and support the person's independence in

activities of daily living, such as dressing, grooming, and meal preparation.

12. Flexibility and Patience: Be flexible and patient in your approach. Activities may need to be adapted based on the individual's current abilities and interests.

13. Meaningful Engagement: Focus on activities that hold personal significance for the individual. For example, gardening, cooking, or caring for a pet can provide a strong sense of purpose.

14. Evaluation and Adaptation: Regularly assess the effectiveness of activities and engagement. Be prepared to adapt activities as the person's needs and abilities change.

15. Safety Considerations: Ensure that activities are safe and suitable for the person's current physical and cognitive abilities. Avoid any activities that could lead to accidents or injuries.

16. Record and Share: Keep a record of the person's favorite activities, preferences, and any positive reactions. Share this information with other

caregivers and family members to ensure consistency in care.

Creating a happy and comfortable life for individuals with dementia through activities and engagement requires a person-centered approach, flexibility, and a commitment to meeting the individual's unique needs. By tailoring activities to the person's interests and abilities, caregivers can provide a sense of purpose, comfort, and joy that greatly enhances the overall quality of life for those living with dementia.

Celebrating Milestones and Special Occasions in Dementia Care

Celebrating milestones and special occasions is a meaningful and enriching aspect of dementia care. These events not only provide moments of joy and connection but also help individuals with dementia maintain a sense of continuity and belonging. Here's an in-depth discussion of the importance of celebrating milestones and special occasions in dementia care:

1. The Significance of Celebration: Celebrations play a crucial role in dementia care by promoting positive emotional experiences, fostering connections with loved ones, and reinforcing a sense of normalcy.

2. Person-Centered Care: Person-centered care is at the heart of celebrating milestones and special occasions. It involves recognizing the individual's unique history, values, and preferences.

3. Identifying Milestones: Milestones can be personal achievements, anniversaries, birthdays, holidays, or significant life events. Identify and celebrate these moments based on the individual's life story.

4. Benefits of Celebrations:
• Celebrations provide numerous benefits, including:
• Creating positive memories and emotional connections.
• Encouraging a sense of accomplishment and self-worth.
• Stimulating cognitive function through reminiscence.

- Combating feelings of isolation and loneliness.
- Rekindling familiar traditions and rituals.

5. Adaptation and Simplification: Depending on the individual's cognitive and physical abilities, adapt and simplify celebrations to ensure they are enjoyable and stress-free. For example, simplify decorations, adjust the guest list, or reduce the duration of the event.

6. Inclusive Celebrations: Include the person with dementia in planning and preparation as much as possible. Their involvement can provide a sense of purpose and participation.

7. Familiar Traditions: Incorporate familiar traditions, customs, and rituals into celebrations. These elements offer a sense of continuity and comfort.

8. Personalized Touch: Personalize celebrations with elements that have significance for the individual, such as favorite foods, music, or activities.

9. Family and Friends: Encourage family and friends to participate in celebrations. These connections can provide emotional support and a sense of belonging.

10. Sensory Engagement: Engage the senses through decorations, music, and sensory-rich elements that evoke positive memories and emotions.

11. Memories and Reminiscence: Create opportunities for reminiscing about past celebrations, sharing stories, and looking through photos or memory books.

12. Calm and Comfort: Maintain a calm and comfortable environment, ensuring that the pace of the celebration aligns with the individual's comfort level.

13. Flexibility: Be flexible in adapting plans if the person with dementia becomes overwhelmed or fatigued during the celebration.

14. Recording Moments: Capture the moments of celebration through photographs or videos to create lasting memories.

15. Record and Share: Keep a record of the individual's favorite milestones and celebrations to share with other caregivers and family members. Consistency in maintaining traditions and rituals can be comforting.

16. Safety and Supervision: Ensure that safety measures are in place during celebrations, such as clear walkways and easy access to restrooms.

Celebrating milestones and special occasions in dementia care is about honoring the person's history and creating positive experiences. By following a person-centered approach, adapting celebrations to the individual's needs, and involving family and friends, caregivers can create meaningful and joyous moments that enhance the overall quality of life for individuals with dementia. These celebrations help maintain connections to the past, boost self-esteem, and foster a sense of belonging despite the challenges of dementia.

Chapter 16

Maintaining a Sense of Dignity in Dementia Care

Maintaining a sense of dignity is a fundamental aspect of providing respectful and compassionate dementia care. Individuals living with dementia often face challenges to their sense of self and autonomy. Here's an in-depth discussion of the importance of maintaining dignity in dementia care:

1. The Significance of Dignity:
Dignity is an intrinsic aspect of being human. For individuals with dementia, preserving their dignity is vital for their emotional well-being and quality of life.

2. Person-Centered Care: Person-centered care forms the foundation of maintaining dignity. This approach recognizes the individual's uniqueness, values, and preferences.

3. Respect for Autonomy: Fostering a sense of autonomy and choice is crucial. Encouraging individuals with dementia to participate in decision-making when possible is a significant aspect of maintaining dignity.

4. Communication: Effective communication is central to preserving dignity. Caregivers should engage in respectful, clear, and empathetic communication. This includes active listening and understanding non-verbal cues.

5. Involvement in Care: Encourage individuals with dementia to actively participate in their care as much as their abilities allow. Involvement in daily activities, self-care, and decision-making helps maintain a sense of self-worth.

6. Personalized Care: Tailor care and interactions to the individual's preferences and needs. This might include personal routines, favorite foods, and familiar activities.

7. Respect for Privacy: Ensure that the individual's privacy is respected during personal care tasks. Use

appropriate strategies to maintain modesty and dignity.

8. Adapt to Changing Abilities: Be adaptable and understanding as the person's cognitive and physical abilities change. Adjust care approaches accordingly while focusing on preserving dignity.

9. Validation and Empathy: Validate the person's emotions and experiences, even if they may not fully comprehend reality. Offering empathy and understanding can ease distress and maintain a sense of dignity.

10. Choice and Control: Offer choices whenever possible. Individuals with dementia should have the opportunity to make decisions, even simple ones, to maintain a sense of control.

11. Avoid Rushing: Give the person ample time to complete tasks and express themselves. Rushing can lead to frustration and a loss of dignity.

12. Sensory Comfort: Create a comfortable environment that addresses sensory needs. This

includes appropriate lighting, comfortable clothing, and temperature control.

13. Encourage Independence: Promote independence in daily activities like dressing, grooming, and eating. Offer support only when necessary to maintain a sense of self-sufficiency.

14. Acknowledge Achievements: Celebrate and acknowledge even small achievements. Recognizing these accomplishments can boost self-esteem and a sense of dignity.

15. Avoid Patronizing Language: Refrain from using condescending or patronizing language when communicating with individuals with dementia. Treat them with the same respect you would offer to anyone else.

16. Inclusive Social Interactions: Foster social interactions and connections with family and friends. Maintaining these relationships can enhance a sense of identity and self-worth.

17. Promote Positive Self-Image: Encourage positive self-image by sharing affirmations,

compliments, and reinforcing the individual's strengths and abilities.

18. End-of-Life Dignity: When reaching the end of life, it's essential to provide comfort and maintain dignity through palliative and end-of-life care.

Preserving a sense of dignity in dementia care requires a person-centered, empathetic, and adaptable approach. It involves empowering individuals with dementia to make choices and participate in their care, while respecting their autonomy and personal preferences. Effective communication, validation, and a focus on positive self-image are key components in fostering dignity despite the challenges of dementia.

Preserving Independence in Dementia Care

Preserving independence is a crucial aspect of providing respectful and person-centered dementia care. Individuals living with dementia often face a decline in their cognitive and physical abilities, but it is essential to empower them to maintain a sense of autonomy and self-worth. Here's an in-depth discussion of the importance of preserving independence in dementia care:

1. The Significance of Independence: Independence is a fundamental aspect of an individual's identity and well-being. For those with dementia, preserving independence can lead to improved self-esteem and overall quality of life.

2. Person-Centered Care: Person-centered care forms the basis for preserving independence. This approach recognizes the individual's unique needs, values, and preferences.

3. Encourage Active Participation: Encourage individuals with dementia to actively participate in their care as much as their abilities allow. Involvement in daily activities, decision-making, and goal-setting helps maintain a sense of control and self-worth.

4. Respect for Autonomy: Fostering autonomy means respecting an individual's right to make choices and decisions, even if they have cognitive

impairments. It is crucial to offer choices whenever possible.

5. Tailored Care Plans: Customize care plans to align with the individual's strengths and abilities. Ensure that care approaches are adapted as cognitive and physical capabilities change over time.

6. Simplicity and Clarity: Keep instructions and tasks simple and easy to understand. Offer clear and concise information, and use visual cues when necessary to enhance comprehension.

7. Routines and Familiarity: Maintain familiar routines and surroundings to minimize confusion and anxiety. Consistency in daily activities can enhance a sense of independence.

8. Avoid Overstimulation: Create a calm and uncluttered environment that minimizes sensory overload. This can help individuals focus on tasks and feel more in control.

9. Time and Patience: Be patient and allow plenty of time for individuals to complete tasks or make

decisions. Avoid rushing, as it can lead to frustration and loss of independence.

10. Adaptive Devices: Implement adaptive devices or technologies that can aid in independent living, such as memory aids, safety features, and communication devices.

11. Empowerment Through Familiar Activities: Encourage engagement in familiar activities and hobbies that the person enjoys. This can boost self-esteem and maintain a sense of identity and purpose.

12. Encourage Self-Care: Promote independence in daily self-care activities, including dressing, grooming, and personal hygiene. Provide support only when necessary.

13. Supportive and Flexible Caregiving: Caregivers should offer support that preserves the individual's autonomy. This means providing assistance only when needed and offering choices whenever possible.

14. Continual Assessment: Continually assess the individual's cognitive and physical abilities, adapting care plans and activities accordingly to promote ongoing independence.

15. Safety Measures: Balance independence with safety. Ensure that the environment is secure, with appropriate safety measures in place to prevent accidents.

16. Acknowledge Achievements: Acknowledge and celebrate the individual's achievements, no matter how small. This recognition boosts self-esteem and reinforces a sense of independence.

17. Inclusive Social Interactions: Encourage social interactions and connections with family and friends. These relationships can provide emotional support and help maintain a sense of belonging.

Preserving independence in dementia care is essential for an individual's self-esteem and overall well-being. It involves empowering individuals to make choices, participate in their care, and continue engaging in activities they enjoy. A person-centered and flexible approach, combined with patience and support, can go a long way in fostering a sense of autonomy and dignity despite the challenges of dementia.

Conclusion

A Compassionate Journey: Reflections on the Caregiver's Journey

Caring for a loved one with dementia is a challenging, often emotional, and deeply compassionate journey. The caregiver's role is significant in providing support, comfort, and maintaining the dignity and well-being of the individual with dementia. In this journey, caregivers have to reflect on the following:

Celebrating Successes:

Caregivers deserve recognition and celebration for their dedication and hard work in the journey of dementia care. Recognizing and celebrating successes, no matter how small, is essential for the caregiver's well-being.

Acknowledging Achievements:

Celebrate the achievements of the individual with dementia. These may be daily tasks, moments of joy, or milestones in their journey.

Self-Appreciation:
Caregivers should acknowledge their own accomplishments. Providing care, maintaining patience, and offering love are significant achievements that deserve recognition.

Finding Joy in Small Moments:
Celebrate the small, joyful moments that occur in the midst of challenging times. These moments often hold profound meaning.

Support and Recognition:
Seek support from family, friends, or support groups who understand the caregiver's journey and can provide recognition and encouragement.

Embracing the Journey Ahead:
The caregiver's journey in dementia care is ongoing, and embracing the path ahead is essential. Here are key aspects to consider:

Self-Care:

Prioritize self-care. Caregivers must care for themselves to continue providing effective care. This involves physical health, emotional well-being, and finding moments for relaxation.

Seek Support:
Continue seeking emotional support and practical assistance from others, such as family, friends, or professional caregivers. Caregivers don't have to navigate the journey alone.

Adaptability:
Recognize that the caregiving journey may change as the individual's needs evolve. Adapt to new circumstances with an open heart and a willingness to modify care strategies.

Resilience:
Embrace resilience as a caregiver. The journey may present challenges, but resilience allows caregivers to face these challenges with strength and determination.

Future Planning:
Consider future plans for the individual's care, such as exploring long-term care options, if necessary.

Making plans in advance helps reduce anxiety and uncertainty.

Emotional Well-Being:
Focus on emotional well-being by seeking therapy or counseling if needed. Taking care of oneself emotionally is essential when providing care.

Gratitude:
Practice gratitude for the meaningful moments and experiences encountered on the caregiving journey. Gratitude can provide perspective and positivity.

Cherish Moments:
Cherish the moments of connection and love between the caregiver and the individual with dementia. These moments are precious and deeply meaningful.

The caregiver's journey in dementia care is marked by compassion, dedication, and love. Celebrating successes, whether big or small, is essential for recognizing the caregiver's efforts and maintaining a positive outlook. Embracing the journey ahead involves self-care, adaptability, and resilience, as the path may change over time. Caregivers should continue to seek support, both emotionally and practically, and remember that the journey, though challenging, is filled with moments of love, connection, and deep meaning.

Resources and References

Caring for individuals with dementia is a complex and demanding task, and caregivers need access to valuable resources and references to provide the best care possible. Here's an overview of the resources and references that can be of assistance in dementia care:

Organizations and Support Services

1. Alzheimer's Association: The Alzheimer's Association is a leading organization dedicated to supporting individuals and families affected by Alzheimer's and other dementias. They offer educational resources, support groups, and a 24/7 helpline.

2. Dementia Caregiver Support Groups: Numerous local and online support groups exist for dementia caregivers. Through these groups, one can meet and exchange experiences with others going through similar struggles.

3. Caregiver Respite Programs: Many communities offer respite programs that provide temporary relief for caregivers, allowing them to recharge while ensuring their loved ones are cared for by professionals.

4. Home Health Services: Home health services offer assistance with medical care, therapy, and personal care needs, allowing individuals with dementia to remain at home while receiving essential support.

5. Adult Day Care Centers: Adult day care centers provide a safe and engaging environment for individuals with dementia during the day, offering a break for caregivers.

Further Reading and References:

* Books:

Several authoritative books offer in-depth information on dementia care. Among the noteworthy books is "The 36-Hour Day" authored by Nancy L. Mace and Peter V. Rabins, "Creating

Moments of Joy" by Jolene Brackey, and "Still Alice" by Lisa Genova.

* Academic and Medical Journals:

Academic journals like the "Journal of Alzheimer's Disease" and "Dementia: The International Journal of Social Research and Practice" provide access to the latest research and findings in the field of dementia care.

* Online Resources:

Reputable websites and online platforms, including the Alzheimer's Association website, Mayo Clinic, and the National Institute on Aging, offer a wealth of information, articles, and guides on dementia care.

* Government Resources:

Government agencies such as the U.S. National Institute on Aging (NIA) and the Centers for Disease Control and Prevention (CDC) provide reliable information, statistics, and guidelines on dementia and caregiving.

* Caregiver Manuals and Guides:

Manuals and guides tailored to dementia caregivers, often available online or through healthcare providers, offer practical tips and strategies for daily care.

* Professional Consultation:

Consulting with healthcare professionals, such as geriatric specialists, psychologists, and social workers, can provide personalized guidance and resources based on the individual's unique needs.

* Dementia Research Institutions:

Research institutions specializing in dementia, such as the Alzheimer's Disease Research Center (ADRC) and the Lewy Body Dementia Association, publish research findings and offer resources for caregivers and families.

* Local Health Services:

Local healthcare providers, hospitals, and clinics may offer resources, referrals, and educational materials specific to dementia care in the community.

These resources and references play a crucial role in equipping caregivers with the knowledge, support, and tools needed to provide effective care for individuals with dementia. Whether seeking emotional support, medical information, or practical caregiving advice, caregivers can find valuable assistance from these sources to enhance the quality of care and improve the lives of those living with dementia.

www.ingramcontent.com/pod-product-compliance
Lightning Source LLC
Chambersburg PA
CBHW050806260726
48660CB00004B/1284